Love lives of the famous

Love lives of the famous

A physician's reflections

Robert B. Greenblatt

B.A., M.D., C.M. (McGill)
Docteur Honoris Causa (Bordeaux)
Professor Emeritus, Department of Endocrinology,
Medical College of Georgia,
Augusta

MTP

Available in USA and Canada from:
J. B. Lippincott Company
East Washington Square
Philadelphia. Pennsylvania 19105

Published by
MTP Press Limited
St. Leonard's House,
Lancaster, England

ISBN: 0 85200 196–7

Photoset, printed and bound
in Great Britain by
REDWOOD BURN LIMITED
Trowbridge & Esher

To Gwenith—my lovely wife,
to whom
William Lyon Mackenzie King, Prime Minister of Canada,
once remarked,
'I've never encountered such beauty in any individual.'

Contents

Acknowledgements

Some of these essays have been published by the author in various journals and I wish to express my gratitude for permission to use much of the material for the following chapters: for Napoleon, Casanova, Mussolini and Goering to *Medical Aspects of Human Sexuality*; for Benjamin Franklin to *Geriatrics*; for Thomas Jefferson to *Medical Opinion*; for Gregory Pincus to *MedCom*; and for King David to J. B. Lippincott Company, from my book *Search the Scriptures: Modern Medicine and Biblical Personages*.

I wish to acknowledge the help of Mrs Martha Bell and Mrs Karin Fischer for research assistance, and to Mrs Cecilia Farmer and Mrs Ann Booker for their efforts in preparing the manuscripts. I am indebted to Count Clemens De Baillou for revealing to me much about Hitler and Goering, and to the publishers for their co-operation, guidance and encouragement.

Foreword

Modern scientific knowledge and technology have been increasingly used in recent years to illuminate the past, to fill in gaps, revise dates and re-analyze events. A combination of carbon dating and dendrochronology has yielded a mass of new and more accurate information, not just on dates and time-scales but on climatic conditions prevailing during the growth period of individual tree-rings. At the same time, core samples from the seabed and from different earth strata have allowed pollen analysis and offered other evidence, which has given us a far clearer picture of the flora and fauna right into the distant past.

Obviously modern medicine used retrospectively can also give us some fascinating insights into people and events and motivations. Robert Greenblatt was one of the first doctors to realize and make use of this. He is one of the world's great endocrinologists but he is also a gynæcologist and a pathologist. As anyone who knows him will testify, he also happens to be a very good psychologist, and he used knowledge and skills from all these different disciplines in his first book of this kind, *Search the Scriptures*, now in its 20th printing. In that book he applied modern diagnostic techniques and medical knowledge to various biblical characters and events.

In this new book he uses the same shrewd but compassionate blend of medical and psychological insight to examine the sex lives and love lives (not necessarily synonymous) of some famous and infamous people. The sexual aberrations of Hitler and Goering have long been known, but now they are explained in medical and psychiatric terms. People, of course, make history, and so as hormonal or other diseases affect people and their behavior, so also they affect history. We all know the fate of the world might have been different if Cleopatra's nose had been a fraction of an inch longer. But would it also have been different if Napoleon had not suffered from hemorrhoids and what Robert Greenblatt convincingly diagnoses as pituitary gland failure, leading to the fatal lethargy and lack of initiative which lost him the battle of Waterloo?

In 1974, researching for my own book *No Change* on hormone replacement therapy, I met Robert Greenblatt for the first time. I arrived in Augusta, Georgia, where he lives and works, the night before he was due as President of The American Geriatrics Society to lecture at and chair a big conference on the Management of Ageing. With doctors flying in from all over America, with his own house-guests and his own lectures scheduled, I remember wondering how on earth he would find any time for me at all. I was soon to find out. Before 8.30 am on my first morning he was at my hotel to join me and other doctors for a working breakfast. This energy and dynamism was just as evident in the days that followed when, with their permission, I was able to watch him at work among patients in his Clinic. It all spilled over to build around him a charisma from which his patients clearly drew immense confidence. But alongside his medical skills, and very much part and parcel of his approach and his treatment, was a deep psychological insight and a deep compassion for the human condition.

It is these same gifts now which are utilized in this book and in his approach to the famous people he deals with. In a sense they become his patients from the past, but in his gentle hands neither history nor the people who made it are trivialized or diminished.

WENDY COOPER
Sutton Coldfield,
England

Introduction

What forces encourage sexual adventurism in so many world leaders? Can aggressiveness in the body politic equate with sexual aggressiveness? Recent studies in the monkey indicate that as status increases, so does production of sex hormones. Thus, there is an indirect relationship between leadership and hormonal levels. Can the increased levels of androgens be responsible for diversions in the psychosexual sphere? Do the augmented testosterone levels trigger uncontrollable urges for more material success or competitive triumphs? How does the endocrinologist or the social anthropologist explain the excessive and sometimes bizarre sexual activities of individuals who have influenced the tides of history, such as King David, Alexander the Great, Julius Caesar, Charlemagne, Henry VIII, Catherine the Great, Napoleon and many others? Mankind has benefited or has been harmed by the benevolence or the malevolence of its famous and infamous leaders. Many have had obsessive drives. Some were psychotic (Nero), sadistic (Torquemada), paranoic (Stalin), sexually manic (Mussolini) or sadomasochistic (Hitler).

In reviewing the sex lives of some famous and infamous people one might ask: Why was their sexual behavior frequently so startlingly different and often so utterly at variance with their exalted position? Could it be that fame and fortune nurture greater liberties and dimensions in sexual comportment? Power, after all, is the ultimate aphrodisiac. Catherine the Great's sexuality knew no bounds once she became Empress of all the Russias. The struggle for dominance, it appears, is linked with excessive sexual drive which increases dramatically with success.

Sexual behavior is studied with difficulty in man because of the modifying influences of the psyche, environmental stresses, state of nutrition, constitutional illness, neurological and metabolic factors, as well as hormonal status. It is easier to study animals and sub-human species, though extrapolations are not always valid. In observing colonies of rhesus monkeys, one finds that leadership is associated with elevation in male hormone (testosterone) levels in the blood. The question comes to mind as to whether the high

11

androgen levels lead to aggressive behavior or whether the reverse is true. At least in the rhesus species the 'boss' or alpha monkey is always a male. The key to victory is not necessarily sheer physical prowess but status in the colony. Removal from leadership results in a fall of testosterone levels. As a monkey's status increases or diminishes, so does his production of hormones. According to sociobiologist Irwin Bernstein of the Yerkes Research Primate Center in Atlanta, Georgia, 'If you depose a leader, his testosterone level sinks, and if you create a leader, it rises'. Thus leaders are made, not born. The human animal, on the other hand, is far more difficult to fathom. Napoleon, a great leader of men, was sexually and militarily aggressive. His fortunes waned with his declining prowess in the bedroom.

Testosterone levels may be equated not only with sexual behavior but also with social comportment. The gelding of a stallion, the castration of a bull, or the caponizing of a rooster, has a marked taming effect. In the human, however, low or absent androgens may trigger bizarre compensatory behavior as a sort of revenge on the human race. The capon-like Goering may well be representative of such a class of men. In a highly competitive society inadequate males tend to develop hostility toward a socially sanctioned scapegoat. In Hitler's case, it was the Jews. His own economic insecurity, his social inferiority, his lack of gonadal integrity (he had only one testicle), may all have contributed to an ego defect. Prejudice against an ethnic group served as a crutch, bolstered self-esteem, and gave an outlet for destructive impulses born of disappointments earlier in life and repeated failures and frustrations.

Certain leaders, unable to attain the ecstasy of love, seek instead the ecstasy of hatred. Experimentally, certain brain lesions induced in dogs result in states of rage and violence. So too, certain brain lesions (syphilis, tumors, encephalitis), or a deep rooted psychoneurosis, may also produce bestial and sadistic behavior in humans. Stalin for one, and Bishop Torquemada of the Spanish Inquisition for another, may have had brain or mental disturbances to account for their sadism. Aside from neurological and metabolic disorders, sexual behavior is dependent on chromosomal endowment, gonadal integrity, gender identification, childhood rearing, environmental influences and hormonal adequacy. James I, for instance, had trouble with gender identification. Napoleon, as it will be shown, first developed psychogenic impotence and later a hormonal deficiency due to multiple endocrine adenomas. Childhood rearing may have so marred social values for Casanova that by seduction of man, woman and child, he showed his contempt for the human race. The ancient Hebrews considered virility in measuring leadership. When King David 'gat no heat' in being put to the test—bedding Abishag, the beautiful maiden—he abdicated in favor of the virile Solomon— he of a thousand wives.

'The history of the world', Carlyle wrote, 'is but the biography of great men'. I simply write of one aspect in the lives of a few personalities who achieved fame or infamy, and ask: Did fame and power affect their sexual behavior, or did their sexual behavior, in one way or another, influence the events of their day?

ROBERT B. GREENBLATT
Medical College of Georgia
Augusta, Georgia 30902

Chapter 1

The
divine right
of kings

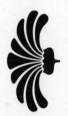

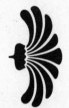

David and Solomon

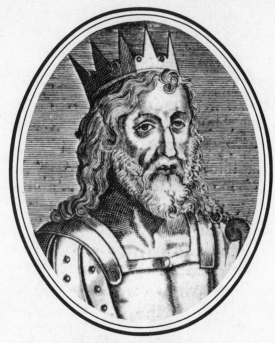

David

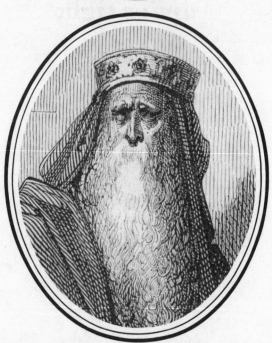

Solomon

King David

None will dispute David's greatness as a king. When a lad, he was gifted in playing the lyre; he exhibited unusual courage as a humble shepherd who slew both lion and bear to protect his father's flocks. A favorite story describes his skill and bravery in killing Goliath, the giant whom he faced alone, armed only with a sling-shot. His sweet songs soothed the sick King Saul, who later became obsessed with jealousy of him. Eventually, David was crowned king over the House of Judah; then, after a long and hard-fought civil war waged against Saul's house, he emerged triumphant to reign over all Israel. His armies succeeded in conquering a feared and hated foe, the Philistines. He captured Jerusalem and made it his capital. The city became the religious and political center of the nation. Displaying adeptness in every way, David was a shrewd military leader, organizer, and administrator. His nature was complex—a common denominator of most geniuses. He affords us a study in personality contrasts—humble but majestic, a sensitive psalmist yet a courageous warrior. Three phases in the love-life of King David are of interest to the student of the human condition.

No Greater Love

David, the young hero, was an accomplished musician. He was brought to the royal court to soothe the king's melancholy and ease his anguish (I *Samuel* 16:14). There he became acquainted with and was befriended by King Saul's son, Jonathan. A true and abiding friendship developed—deep, intense and genuine, and 'Saul's son delighted much in David' (I *Samuel* 19:1). The relationship exemplified a love greater and more ennobling than that between man and woman, for it was brotherly love in its highest sense—'The soul of Jonathan was knit with the soul of David, and Jonathan loved him as his own soul' (I *Samuel* 18:1).

The attraction between the two has been seized upon by some as an example of homosexual love. On learning that Jonathan perished in battle, David lamented: 'I am distressed for thee, my brother Jonathan; very pleasant hast thou been unto me, thy love to me was wonderful, passing the love of women'. For many scholars, the high praise accorded the love between these two youths was reminiscent of the spirit that pervades Plato's Symposium. The Greeks found beauty magnetic without respect to sex, and many amongst them believed that there was no higher form of love than homosexual love. However, the insinuation that the tender companionship of David and Jonathan was anything other than spiritual is without foundation. The whole affair reminds one of the accusation that William Shakespeare was homosexual because of lines found in many of his sonnets which exhalt a man's love for another man. By such lines as 'But since she prick't thee out for women's pleasure Mine by thy love, and thy love's use their treasure' (*Sonnet 20*), or 'Two loves I have . . . the better angel is a man right fair' (*Sonnet 144*), he was merely showing his heartfelt appreciation to his patron. Nonetheless, Oscar Wilde, trenchant homosexual, used these and other lines to impugn the Bard of Avon. Homosexuals have done their utmost to annexe Shakespeare and use him as an advertisement of their own peculiarity. So too has the ennobling friendship of David and Jonathan been misinterpreted and beclouded by lascivious and professional debunkers. David was a sentimental man who loved greatly and felt deeply. When his son Absalom was killed in armed rebellion against him, this sentimentality came to the fore. In his grief, he wailed, 'would God I had died for thee, O Absalom, my son, my son!'

Lustful Love

King David had problems born of the struggle of opposing instincts within himself. He was a man who cherished a specially close contact with God: from his simple faith had grown a strong, unbending conscience; and he was a man of great passion as well, having taken eight wives and ten concubines as permitted under the law. Within him, his conscience was now to struggle with his passion become lust, and worse.

At fifty he succumbed to a temptation that was to bring sore trouble. At this age, we realize, a man may be tempted to prove his virility simply because he has less of it, because his sexuality has diminished. It is a time of life when physical, mental, and emotional upsets are not endured easily. Resistance is low; a surge of restlessness, of loneliness, is a constant threat. David had returned to his palace, after numerous victories, for relaxation well earned. Restive, he 'arose from off his bed, and walked upon the roof of the king's house: and from the roof he saw a woman washing herself; and the woman was very beautiful to look upon'. She was Bathsheba, wife of Uriah, one of David's brave and loyal captains. A sudden desire subdued David's sense of righteousness and impulsively he sent for her. She, doubtless flattered to be summoned by her king, submitted to his advances. When she discovered herself pregnant, David lost no time in bringing her husband home from the battle, expecting, thereby, to conceal his adultery. But Uriah, despite all persuasion, refused to enter his house while Israel's army suffered on the grim field of battle. Sending Uriah back to the fighting, David had him placed in a position where death was inescapable, and, after the days of mourning, he took Bathsheba to be his wife. The Bathsheba affair could not be dismissed as mere lust abetted by royal prerogative, for the relationship turned out to be an enduring one. Bathsheba was his favorite wife. Nevertheless, the effect of this tragic affair on a sensitive, God-loving man who had sought to live in righteousness cannot be overestimated. David had lost contact with his Lord, and no longer understood himself. Men of his character are prone to expect trouble; they might even invite it as penance to soothe their feelings of guilt.

And trouble came, announced by Nathan the prophet: 'Wherefore hast thou despised the commandment of the Lord, to do evil in his sight? thou hast killed Uriah the Hittite with the sword, and has taken his wife to be thy wife, . . . Now therefore the sword shall never depart from thine house; . . . Thus saith the Lord, Behold, I will raise up evil against thee' (II *Samuel* 12:9–11).

David had expected grim punishment, and Nathan's unstill voice foreshadowed his soul's agony. He suffered one misfortune after another, and his personal concerns gave him harsher trial than many overwhelming national problems. Certain that his woes were a sure sign of God's wrath, the once-majestic king aged beyond his years—his feelings of guilt played havoc with his well-being, and he could never forget Nathan's renunciation, 'Thou art the man'.

Love's Labor Lost

From the age of fifty, King David had no rest from misfortune and emotional turmoil. At seventy, he was so spent that he could lead his people no longer. Was he suffering from circulatory failure due to arteriosclerosis, severe anemia, hypothyroidism, or from general apathy and decrepitude? Rumblings were abroad, rumor raced through the kingdom that the king was finished, and his son Adonijah laid claim to the throne.

The criterion that determined the king's loss of usefulness to his state seems strange to us. Was the fact that he 'gat no heat' when covered with clothes a valid test of his fitness for leadership? The clinical observation was not strong enough to force his abdication; a more exacting test was needed, and the Israelites were prone to equate sexual prowess with virility and strength.

'Wherefore his servants said unto him, Let there be sought for my lord the king a young virgin: and let her stand before the king, and let her cherish him, and let her lie in thy bosom, that my lord the king may get heat.'

'So they sought for a fair damsel throughout all the coasts of Israel, and found Abishag a Shunammite, and brought her to the king.'

'And the damsel was very fair, and cherished the king, and ministered to him: but the king knew her not' (I *Kings* 1:2–4).

What pride must have been in the hearts of Abishag's parents when their daughter was chosen from all Israel to lie with the king. Although the origin of this sanctioned privilege is lost in antiquity, the claim of a prince continued through the middle ages. *Le droit de seigneur* could not be denied the lord of a domain, a baron, or the prince of a petty principality. The custom was extended to rights on the wedding night of the bride, and *droit de noce* often was exacted from subjugated people.

When Abishag tried to arouse the king, he still 'gat no heat' and so failed the test—love's labor lost. One can imagine her proud and anxious parents awaiting her return, their meeting, and the disillusion and dismay of all three. Word of the king's loss of virility spread throughout the kingdom, and his leadership was in doubt. Bathsheba confronted the king to ensure that he declare Solomon, her son by him, as successor. David named him to ascend the throne, advancing him over other brothers who outranked him in seniority and experience.

We may wonder whether David was in the throes of the male climacteric, akin to the female change of life. Although students of glandular physiology have not been of unanimous opinion that the male climacteric exists, evidence that it does is strong. We know today that the climacteric occurs in both sexes, but that it affects only a small portion of men. With advancing years, testicular androgens lessen considerably. Testicular decline is great in some and less in others. Newer studies of serum testosterone (the male hormone) levels in aging males reveal that there is indeed a steady decline from the age of fifty onwards. However, some men maintain sexual virility well into old age and their testosterone values may equal those of men of twenty-five. Surprisingly, peripheral serum estradiol (the female hormone) levels in aged men are comparable to those found in postmenopausal women.

Environmental and emotional factors play important roles and can hasten senescence. An early indication of the male climacteric is loss of ability to concentrate, irritability and melancholia. At this stage, men often become antisocial and many lose confidence in their abilities. By the age of seventy, the lamp of life and love was dimmed for David, the majestic king who had lived life to the fullest, loved greatly, and suffered much.

King Solomon

'Be thou strong therefore, and shew thyself a man' (I Kings 2:2).

Thus did David, on his deathbed, charge his son Solomon. And Solomon acted accordingly: he ruthlessly eliminated the opposition by assassination and ruled the kingdom for the next forty years with a firm hand. Solomon followed in the footsteps of his righteous father—he at whom Nathan the Prophet had pointed an accusing finger in the Bathsheba affair, saying 'Thou art the man'. Properly chastised, David henceforth led a life dedicated to the Lord, and Solomon his son did likewise—for a time.

On Solomon's succession to the kingship, he secured his dynasty by espousing the Pharaoh's daughter, thus protecting his southern borders. He secured his northern borders by extending and implementing the existing alliance with Hiram, the ruler of Tyre. He developed friendly relations with the various neighboring countries by marrying their princesses. In this manner he consolidated his kingdom and, by assuring a measure of peace, was able to devote his energies to a vast building program, to promotion of commerce, and to establishing a respected place for Israel among the nations.

Solomon was a shrewd judge of character; his keen worldly wit and winning personality endeared him to the people. He won a reputation for remarkable wisdom and, as usual, time and circumstance conspired to magnify his accomplishments. Emissaries and kings from abroad brought gifts of precious stones as they came to pay him homage, to savor his wise sayings, and to learn of his ways. Even the Queen of Sheba journied to Jerusalem 'with a very great train, with camels that bare spices, and very much gold, and precious stones: and when she was come to Solomon, she communed with him of all that was in his heart' (I *Kings* 10:2). The Bible relates that Solomon gave unto the Queen of Sheba all her desire, whatever she asked. I am given to wonder whether the passage in the Song of Solomon is a reference to the Queen of Sheba, the Ethiopian—'Let him kiss me with kisses of his mouth; for thy love is better than wine . . . the king hath brought me into his chambers . . . I am black, but comely' (1:2,4,5).

As to Solomon's wisdom, the Bible tells that 'he spake three thousand proverbs'; as to his poetic ability, 'his songs were a thousand and five'. The Lord gave Solomon 'a wise and understanding heart'. He demonstrated these qualities when he ordered a living child to be cut in two, giving half to each of two women who claimed the infant as her own. The true mother revealed herself when she begged the king not to slay the child but to give it to the other woman.

Solomon was a great pragmatist. He built a merchant fleet and, in partnership with Hiram, his ships carried on extensive commerce not only from Mediterranean ports but also from the port at the head of the Gulf of Akaba for traffic with Arabia. There was a considerable trade in horses; his imports were on a grand scale, his vessels 'bringing gold, and silver, ivory, and apes, and peacocks' (I *Kings* 10:22). Solomon brought Israel fully into the currents of culture and commerce. Jerusalem became a city of wealth and luxury.

Solomon was determined to modernize his country: he rebuilt cities in the pattern of his more prosperous neighbors, constructed market places and storage houses. But taking precedence over all was the building of the most lavish royal dwelling in the Middle East—an undertaking that took thirteen years and a good part of the country's treasury. The palace was splendidly built and sumptuously appointed. Next was the erection of a temple that would be a tribute to the majesty of his God. It was magnificent. The massive blocks of stone were hewn from the quarries outside Jerusalem, the wooden adornments and structural parts were of stately cedars brought in from Lebanon. Then the military presence was made apparent not only to forestall discontent and revolt but so that Judah and Israel could dwell in safety, 'every man under his vine and under his fig tree from Dan to Beer-sheba'. This required twelve thousand horsemen and fourteen hundred chariots. Barracks were built for the horsemen, stables for the horses, arsenals for the chariots and implements of war. He built a protective wall around Jerusalem and fortified the cities on the borders.

Solomon was a sensuous and pleasure-seeking man. He had many queens and concubines for whom he constructed elaborate and splendid houses and a luxurious harem. Many of his marriages were politically inspired. He loved many strange women, including the daughter of Pharaoh, and women of the Moabites, Ammonites, Edomites, Zidoneans, and Hittites. He had seven hundred wives and princesses and three hundred concubines. To feed, entertain, and clothe this multitude was a prodigious undertaking.

Admittedly, Solomon brought fame and fortune to little Israel—but at a price! His prodigality was inordinate; his court, costly; the maintenance of his peace-time army, exorbitant; the upkeep of his harem, an extravagance; the cost of the palatial dwellings and temple, ruinous. The taxes that were levied impoverished the rank and file of the people. The chronicler of the book of Kings remarks with a suspicion of bitterness, 'all of King Solomon's drinking vessels were of pure gold; none were of silver'.

Another picture of Solomon emerges from the study of this 'wise' ruler. The pomp and glitter of his court remind one of the saying, 'all is vanity'. His palace and even the temple are, in reality, monuments to his ego. Little wonder that at a later date, Jesus was able to make the cynical comparison, 'Consider the lilies of the field, how they grow; they toil not, neither do they spin: and yet I say unto you, That even Solomon in all his glory was not arrayed like one of these' (*Matthew* 6:28,29). Solomon was a sensualist— the very idea of a thousand wives and concubines is a conceit, the enormity of which is beyond belief. Yet he was a sensitive man with a poetic flare. With or without the singing of the birds, and the voice of the turtledove in the land, the *Song of Solomon* proclaimed with more charm than innocence his preoccupation with the female breast: 'Thy two breasts are like two young roes that are twins, which feed among the lilies. Until the day break, and the shadows flee away, I will get me to the mountain of myrrh, and to the hill of frankincense' (4:5,6).

The *Song of Solomon* has been dismissed by some as both pagan and lewd. Such pious dissaproval of a theme written with delicacy and tenderness nearly resulted in exclusion of this classic of literature from the Bible. Even at the close of the last century, the

Reverend E. P. Eddruff, Prebendary of Salisbury Cathedral, admonished that 'such a book as the *Song of Solomon* may not be fitted for public reading in a mixed congregation, or even in private reading by the pure of heart'. Despite such protestations, the Song will remain a pæan to love, in praise of the body beautiful, and a timeless tribute to womanhood.

What of the man himself? Solomon was particularly relentless toward the opponents of his succession. A number of military leaders who had supported his brother Adonijah's candidacy for the throne were slain without the formality of a pretext. He started his reign as a petty despot and continued to rule with unmistakable sternness. Though he was counted by tradition as the wisest of his time, the clever master of phrases was a most harsh master of men.

Many modern critics describe him as the despoiler of his people, and his life, one long extravagance. Abram Leon Sachar, in *A History of the Jews,* feels that the criticism is unfair, for Solomon:

> opened the Hebrew world to new and far-reaching influences. He expanded the cultural boundaries of Israel. The price was perhaps too high; too many backs were bent and too many purses drained to pay for the royal projects. But they helped to enrich the narrow life of Israel as much as they helped to satisfy the vanity of the king.

He was a pleasure-loving monarch. While his people groaned under the burden of heavy taxes, he lived riotously and luxuriated in his harem. The *Song of Solomon* mentions 'sixty queens and eighty concubines and virgins without number'. It was the women who were responsible for his real downfall: 'When Solomon was old, his wives turned away his heart after other gods: and his heart was not perfect with the Lord his God, as was the heart of David his father' (I *Kings* 11:4). Solomon fell under the influence of his foreign wives and to appease them he erected altars to alien dieties, and participated in their pagan rites. So long as Solomon kept the faith, the rank and file were willing to endure and excuse the heavy taxes because of national pride. But his departure from orthodoxy shocked and utterly displeased the people and discontent grew. Rumblings and rebellion were heard throughout the land. On his death, ten tribes rebelled and set up their own Kingdom of Israel, leaving the remaining two tribes to hold dominion over Jerusalem and its environs, the Kingdom of Judea. The grandeur of Solomon's works came to naught.

Solomon, the Wise, a slave to voluptuousness, was victimized by the women in his life. Throughout the history of mankind, it appears that great leaders have been heir to this grievous fault. When the grand monarch died, his obituary was no glowing testimonial, for the chronicler charitably notes, he 'went not fully after the Lord, as did David his father'.

Chapter 2

The strange affinities of two of the kings of England

Richard I and James I

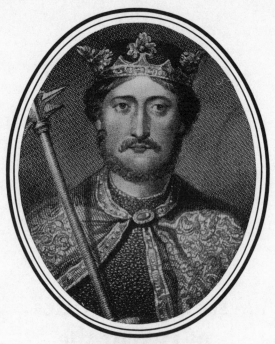

Richard I

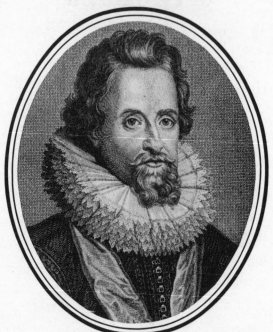

James I

Richard the Lion-hearted

In studying the social and private lives of the monarchs of England, the surprising fact emerges that at least six of them had a strange proclivity for members of their own sex. James Graham, in his book *The Homosexual Kings of England*, reveals the names of William II, Richard I, Edward II, Richard II, James I and William III. Only William II was purely homosexual, untainted by any woman; the others were bisexual.

Male homosexuality has been prevalent in England since the Norman Conquest. In Norman England, long-haired effeminate youths mimicked women in extravagant dress and mannerisms. E. A. Freeman, biographer of William II, wrote 'Into the details of his private life it is well not to grope too narrowly. In him England might see on her own soil habits of the ancient Greek . . .'. Homosexuality had become a *modus vivendi*. The sin had become so public that hardly anyone took notice of it, so that William II could write to a favorite (a euphemism for homosexual partner), 'It seems to me a most extraordinary thing that one may not feel regard and affection for a young man without it being criminal. . . . Return to me and I shall love you all my life'. In today's England and in several of the countries of Europe, as well as in America, it is said that this deviation from the norm afflicts every tenth man.

Two illustrious Kings of England—one, Richard I, the other, James I—presented two different life-styles. One was a conscience-ridden closet homosexual; the other, a defiant deviate.

Richard I (1157–1199), King of England, was a French nobleman, son of Henry II of France; his mother was the famous Eleanor of Aquitaine. He was nicknamed Coeur de Lion (the Lion-Hearted). A majestic statue stands in the Old Palace Yard of Westminster Abbey as a symbol of a knight-errant king who for the glory of Christ and the Cross fought to win the Holy Land from the Saracens. He is presented as an heroic figure sitting astride his horse with sword uplifted. Richard became heir to the throne of England and Normandy after the death of his elder brother, Henry, the heir apparent with whom he carried on a fratricidal war. His father, Henry II, favored Richard in this struggle and marched to his aid. But just as brother did strive against brother, so did son later strive against father. Obsessively ambitious, he ultimately renounced his own father to gain his ends. He managed to project the image of gallantry and elegance. Though history shows that he was an absentee king who held England in fief to France, he was nonetheless a popular hero.

Richard succeeded to the throne of England in 1183. Upon hearing of Saladin's crushing defeat of the Crusaders, he decided to devote his life to the reconquest of Jerusalem—he took the Cross. To fulfill his crusading vows he sacrificed all other interests and raised the necessary funds by the most reckless means. He put up for auction the highest offices and honors, and by other expedients managed to raise sufficient monies to equip a force of four thousand men-at-arms, and as many foot soldiers, with a fleet of a hundred transports.

For the Christian it was an opportunity to consecrate his fighting instinct. Chivalry directed the layman to defend what was right— the preaching of the Crusaders directed him to attack what was wrong, in other words, the possession of the Sepulchre of Christ by the Mohammedan infidel. It was chivalry on the offense, but the knight who joined the crusaders, under the aegis of the Church, did so more likely than not to attain salvation and remission of sins. The Crusaders, though they touched the summits of daring and devotion, also sank into the deep abyss of shame, self-interest, achievement of riches and acquisition of lands. Pillage, rape, and murder were overlooked or condoned because such happenings were merely incidental to the greater struggle on behalf of the cross. Richard the Lion-Hearted joined the crusading 'armies' in Sicily and remained there during the winter of 1190–1191. Instead of going directly to the aid of the Christian besiegers of Acre he first went on to conquer Cyprus—partly in knight-errantry; partly to avenge an insult to Princess Berengaria, daughter of the King of Navarre, whom he married in Cyprus in May 1191; and partly for profit, for he later sold Cyprus to his ally and fellow crusader, Guy F. Lusignan. Richard finally sailed for Acre, arriving June 8 1191. In spite of dissention in the Christian camp which he helped to foment, and thanks to his energy and skill, he successfully reduced Acre. He remained in the Holy Land for sixteen months winning some important battles and fortifying Jaffa. However, he failed to displace the Mohammedan hold on Jerusalem, perhaps because of his preoccupation with intrigue, quarrels, and political maneuvering. On his voyage of return to England he was captured by Leopold of Austria, whose hostility he had incurred, and was compelled to purchase his release by the payment of a heavy ransom.

The crusades were in fact medieval 'armed' pilgrimages and served several purposes. Aside from salvation and remission of sin, they afforded an opportunity to tour the continent and break away from dull routine. Richard and his knights toured Italy before reaching Messina in Sicily. It was there that Richard, the warrior, felt contrite and guilt-ridden and would not rest until the bishops would hear his confession and give him absolution. It took place in Reginald de Muhec's chapel in Messina before an assembly of bishops and knights. He appeared before them in a plain cloak which he immediately discarded. There he stood naked before them and abased himself while making a confession of homosexuality. He confessed the foulness of his life to God. The bishops pronounced absolution and the king promised not to slip back into sin again. But in spite of those vows, and repeated warnings of the fate of Sodom, Richard did lapse back into his old ways. He later confessed again, did penance, and brought his wife back to his side. The queen was with him in Acre and during his imprisonment in Vienna, but otherwise they went their separate ways.

In medieval times when knighthood was in flower, the gallant knight honored, protected, adored and admired his lady and romanced her with poetry and song. He placed her on a pedestal to be worshipped and not to sully, substituting romantic love for intimacy. For sport, the knights jousted; for sex, they had their wenches; for adventure, they were ready to do battle at the bidding of their seigneur, or lord of the domain to whom they owed their fealty.

The myth of Richard I as the epitome of chivalry, of courtly love, of steadfast devotion to Christendom has been perpetuated because historians have glossed over the darker side of his character. His prodigious energy, courage, chivalric stature and poetic skill cannot be denied. However, he was a bad son, a poor husband, a selfish ruler, a rapacious and vengeful man, and a sodomite who manipulated the Church to absolve him of his carnal sins. He became the undisputed leader of the Third Crusade and devoted his talents to the glory of Christ and the Cross, thereby hoping to gain salvation for his guilt-ridden soul. History proves that Richard by no means embodied the current ideal of chivalrous excellence. His escutcheon is stained by needless acts of cruelty, such as the massacre of over two thousand Saracen prisoners at Acre. As a ruler, he was equally rapacious—not one useful measure can be placed to his credit. He was never happier than when engaged in war. This Third Crusade proved not only a failure but a disaster to the Eastern Christian establishment.

James I

Contrast the elegant Richard I with the crass and coarse Scot, James I (1566–1625), King of England and Ireland, and as James VI, ruler of Scotland. He was the son of Mary Queen of Scots, born in Edinburgh Castle. His tutors gave him a sound education, especially in language and theology, which developed in him literary ambitions rarely found in princes. He expounded views of the nature of royal authority and the divine right of Kings and when he succeeded to the English throne on the death of Elizabeth I (March 14 1603), he had a clearly defined concept of kingship.

While King of Scotland, at twenty-three, he married Princess Anne of Denmark—a marriage made more to secure the dynasty than for love. He had a notorious aversion toward women and a particular affinity for men. When he went to London to claim the crown of England he made a good impression and was well received. He was tall and broad-shouldered; he had a goodly figure and displayed a sense of wit and obvious intelligence. One

of his first important acts was to gather a group of notable theologians to prepare an exact translation of the Holy Scriptures from
the ancient Hebrew and Greek into the English tongue. The
authorized version was completed in 1611 and is unmatched in
English literature for the beauty of its prose. This version remained
unchanged for over 350 years and is still in use by English-speaking
Anglicans and Christian Protestant groups the world over.

The felicity with which these Biblical scholars interpreted
ancient Hebrew manuscripts may be judged by the following: the
passage in the King James Version, 'His breasts are full of milk' (*Job*
21:24) seemed so incredible that it was thought to be erroneous.
Theologians apologetically offered another interpretation such as
found in the Latin Bible, '*Viscera eus sunt adipe plena*' (his viscera are
full of fat), or the French Bible, '*Ses flancs chargés de graisse*' (his
flanks are charged with fat). The Revised Standard Version (RSV)
published in 1942 retrenched from the original and subverted *Job*
21:24 to read, 'His body is full of fat'. Actually, there is no need for
an exegesis of the statement in question for it is also found in the
Geneva Bible of 1560 ('His breasts are full of milke and his bones
run full of marowe'). Some years ago the *Book of Job* was recovered
from Cave XI of Khirbet Qumran in the Judean wilderness. Written in Aramaic over two thousand years ago, it leaves no doubt as
to the meaning of the passage in question, 'His teats are full of
milk'. Recent advances in our knowledge of lactation now offers a
rational explanation as to how psychophysical and endocrine glandular disorders can cause milk to appear in the breasts of man. The
passage in *Job*, as found in the King James Version, was not simply
a figure of speech but an accurate translation.

The nation was grateful for James's great gift to Christendom.
However, once his crown was secure, the true nature of the man
began to unfold. J. B. Kenyon in his book *The Stuarts* said of him,
'at dinners, his vulgarity, obscenity, and uproarious pedantry had
full play, as he slobbered in his drink, cracked bawdy jests, and
swapped texts and references with the ecclesiasts who stood behind
his chair, capping all with a casual blasphemy'. He drank and ate
indiscriminantly. His interior organs were so full that he got rid of

the vast surplus in whatever disgusting fashion—up or down. He once scolded a Presbyterian minister, 'I give not a turd for your preaching'.

James I surrounded himself with brilliant personages. William Harvey was his physician; Francis Bacon, his political adviser; and John Donne attended to his spiritual needs. His wife, Queen Anne, provided him with three offspring. Otherwise, he had little use for her. Along with his love of food and drink, he loved to hunt much of the year with his sexually compatible intimates. Perhaps this obsession with hunting was a ploy to get away as often as possible from the Queen and from the boredom of the Court. The English people hardly knew him and when they complained that they saw little of his face, the King, according to one biographer, replied, 'God's wounds! I'll pull down my breeches and they shall see my arse!'

The English became disillusioned with their King. He, who started off with such promise, was distracted from his sovereign role by pederasty and hard drinking. The Puritans called him a sodomite. All his life he was attracted to handsome men; he had many lovers. It was said that 'the love the King showed them was as amorously conveyed as if he had mistaken their sex and thought them ladies . . . nor was his love carried on with discretion . . .'. He had many favorites and showed no shame or remorse in openly kissing and fawning over them in a most lascivious manner. Though his attachment was to effeminate men, he nonetheless took on some of the mannerisms himself by displaying a feminine fondness for wearing jewels.

The lavish creation of new peers, and later in his reign, his sub-servience to 'favorites' loosened the crown's hold upon the House of Lords. The King succumbed to the influence of one of his cata-mites, the upstart and incompetent Scot, Robert Carr, Earl of Somerset. Scandal involving the Earl broke out and the King was forced to dismiss him. James I, when forty-seven years of age, had a handsome twenty-two-year-old attendant, who became the real love of his life. He was George Villiers. The portrait of this delicate and effeminate man hangs in the National Gallery in London.

James I bestowed upon him every honor possible—Viscount Villiers in 1616, Earl of Buckingham in 1617. The King referred to him as 'sweet child and wife'. Addressing his council in 1617 he said, 'I, James, am neither a god nor an angel but a man like any other. Therefore, I act like a man, and confess to loving those dear to me more than other men. You may be sure I love the Earl of Buckingham more than anyone else, and more than any who are here assembled. I wish to speak in my own behalf and not to have it thought to be a defect, for Jesus Christ did the same and therefore I cannot be blamed. Christ had his John, I have my George'. Two years later he elevated his 'favorite' to Marquis. As the King was aging, he felt the pangs of loneliness and a fear of losing his beloved for he wrote to Villiers 'that I rather live banished in any part of the earth with you, than live a sorrowful widow-life without you'. Twenty-two years after his succession to the throne of England, the ailing King died in fear and misery, incontinent and in filth.

The King was dead. The evil was interred with his bones, the 'good' lives on in the King James Version of the Bible of which he was prime mover and one of the principal authors. He was laid to rest after a magnificent and elaborate funeral amid pæans of praise and torrents of tears and lamentations. The divine right of Kings— what a mockery!

Chapter 3

Hemorrhoids, sex and history

Louis XIV and Napoleon

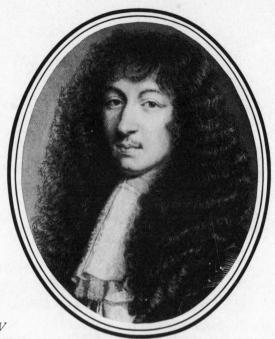

Louis XIV

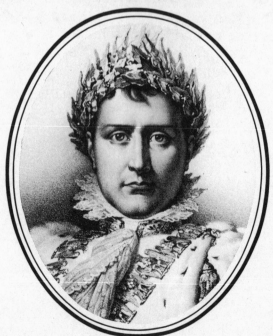

Napoleon

Louis XIV

France enjoyed two great epochs under the leadership of two egotistical men, Louis XIV and Napoleon I. What did these two famous men have in common? Both had numerous love affairs, suffered greatly from hemorrhoids, and both played a monumental role in history.

Louis XIV (1638–1715) was the son of Louis XIII and Anne of Austria. Upon the death of his father in 1643, he was crowned King at the age of five. When the future Louis XIV was born at St Germain-en-Laye, Louis XIII regarded the event with derision, refusing even to kiss the Queen on his visitation to her. Why did the King fail to manifest any pleasure in seeing the infant that was going to perpetuate the dynasty? He was lugubrious because he knew something that she did not know. Yes, he did spend the night with her some nine months previously but he could not father a child. He loved his two current mistresses more than his Queen yet, unlike many another royal favorite, neither bore him any offspring. Was the King impotent or merely sterile? M. Vernadeau, in his book *Le Medicin de la Reyne*, claimed that the physicians who performed the autopsy on Louis XIII declared 'he could not have a child'.

During the minority rule of Louis XIV his mother left the conduct of affairs of state entirely in the hands of her First Minister, Cardinal Mazarin. The Cardinal was the boy's godfather; he was also reputed to be one of the Queen's lovers. Anne of Austria was quite a coquette; she proved an unfaithful wife having had several abortions while living in separation from the King.

Who was the father of Louis XIV? Some thought the honors should go to Mazarin, others suggested Cardinal Richelieu, but Pierre Marteau wrote in his book *Les Amours d'Anne d'Autriche* that Count de la Rivière was the culprit. At any rate, everyone is in accord with the bastardy of the King; putative is the question of fatherhood.

At the age of twenty-one, Louis XIV married his cousin, the Infanta Maria Theresa and soon had a son by her. About this time he was enraptured with his father's hunting lodge and repaired there often, giving parties in the garden for his mistress and a band of young friends. He decided to build a monumental palace on the site, preserving the original lodge—the future Versailles.

On the death of Mazarin, he took complete charge and announced his intention of being his own First Minister. He ruled in a most autocratic manner. Louis XIV was probably the most absolute and egotistical monarch ever to sit on the throne of France. He was an energetic man who personally took charge of every detail in government. His wish was to make his realm the most powerful in Europe, his Court the most brilliant, his palace at Versailles the most magnificent. He was the patron of artists, musicians, and actors, who in turn served to amuse him and the nobility. Indeed, he did succeed for a time and France unquestionably became the first state in Europe, both in arms and in the arts.

Louis XIV had a noble mien: regal to the core, he walked with extraordinary grace, never made an ill-considered gesture. Swarthy in appearance with an aquiline nose and small dark eyes, he had none of the features of the tall and gentle King Louis XIII. Nancy Mitford, in her book *The Sun King*, suggests that he probably had Jewish and Moorish blood in him since he was descended from the royal Aragon family. He was not tall as Mitford depicts him for he was only 1 m 62 cm (5 feet $2\frac{1}{4}$ inches) in height. He was a vain man. Being small of stature, he was, perhaps, the first to introduce elevated shoes, the forerunner of fancy high-heeled footwear so popular today among certain strata of society. This innovation permitted him to appear tall enough so that the seigneurs who visited his Court would not tower over him. He was an ambitious man, but his interests began to change and he turned from contentment with national development to ambitious expansionism at the expense of his European neighbors. Unlike the brave Louis XIII who rushed to do battle with his enemies and to expose himself in combat, Louis XIV went to the wars in a stagecoach to observe the fighting from a comfortable and safe vantage point. He often brought his mistresses with him to view the grand spectacle.

Louis XIV was a frivolous man, and though he worked diligently at being the 'Grand Monarch', nonetheless devoted much time to a life of gaiety, the hunt, and to women. Though his wife, Maria Theresa, bore him children, there was no community of tastes between them and the chief influence at court was not to be found in the Queen but in a succession of avowed mistresses, Louise de la Vallière, the Marquise de Montespan, and Madame de Maintenon.

It was customary for the king of France to have both a wife and a declared mistress who was almost a second wife. As soon as Queen Anne died, Louis XIV immediately recognized Louise de la Vallière as his titular mistress, made her a duchess and legitimized their baby daughter, Maria-Ann. He treated his principal mistresses with considerable consideration, built beautiful houses for them, gave important and lucrative offices to members and relatives of their families. For the Marquise de Montespan and her sister, the Marquise de Thianges (who incidentally also shared his bed on many occasions) Louis XIV obtained a percentage on all the meat and tobacco sold in Paris so that they could have independent fortunes. Louise de la Vallière lost favor with the King and retired to a convent. Mistresses Montespan and Maintenon were worried when the King lost interest in their quarrels over him. Loosening his royal restraints, he was now inclined to go to bed with any woman who was at hand. A series of violent love-affairs followed. In all he had 17 children with his wife and his paramours, but his real love in the autumn of his life was Madame de Maintenon, of whom it is recounted that one day, on meeting the Marquise de Montespan on the Queen's staircase, she remarked in her dry wit, 'You are going down, Madame? I am going up'. The King had apartments for all three women on his own floor. After the Queen's death, he entered into a morganatic marriage with Madame de Maintenon. She was pious, ladylike, and a great comfort to the aging King.

For more than a dozen years, the King was troubled by hemorrhoids and at the age of forty-three developed a fistula-in-ano. His anal preoccupation caused him to become dour and sombre. At about this point in time, whether due to the sobering effect of a painful '*derrière*' or to the pious urging of Madame de Maintenon, he turned away from frivolity and became a religious man. The courtiers reflected the new attitude of the master and each one interested himself in some religious project.

When he was forty-two (a year before the first operation for the correction of his fistula) Louis XIV revoked the Edict of Nantes (1685), the celebrated charter that had granted tolerance to the Protestants known as Huguenots. Persecuted and deprived of their religious and civil liberties, four hundred thousand of the most industrious and finest citizens of France sought refuge in Germany, Holland, and England. Many Huguenots journeyed to America and settled in South Carolina; there they fostered a climate of religious freedom and the realization of the American dream. The strength of France was seriously diminished.

Throughout his reign, as Louis' hemorrhoids grew more painful, his imperious temper grew shorter and his policies became self-defeating. A succession of military operations not only depleted the flower of France but also its exchequer. In the War of the Spanish Succession, Marlborough and his allies defeated Louis' armies and the fortunes of France began to dwindle. Louis XIV's extravagance in building Versailles—the construction of which took twenty years—impoverished the country. He imposed intolerable taxes, was contemptuous of the masses and oblivious to their needs. The seeds were being sown for the bloody revolution that was eventually to erupt. In reflection, who can say to what degree the torment of Louis XIV's affliction or how much the pious pressures from his religiously inclined mistress contributed to bringing mighty France to the brink of ruin after an epoch of ineffable grandeur. It would appear that hemorrhoids and a mistress had a great bearing on his goals and colored his political philosophy and geopolitics.

How great a monarch was Louis XIV, known as the Sun King? The great period which bears his name had already reached its zenith before he began his rule. The King died on September 1 1715, after the longest recorded reign in European history. The judgement of posterity has not repeated the flattering verdict of his contemporaries—*le Roi Soleil*—but as a King, he was every inch a Monarch.

Napoleon Bonaparte

Armo virumque cano—I tell the tale of a great soldier and his sexual denouement. None since Charlemagne left a greater legacy to European history than Napoleon, yet his own love story was one of pathetic failure. He defined love as '*une sottise faite a deux*' (folly for two). Aside from his hemorrhoids and urinary disturbance, did Napoleon's sexual frustrations have a bearing on history?

Since sex colors our entire lives, one may ask in what manner did Napoleon's sex life have a bearing on the pressing and tumultuous happenings of his day? And how, later on, did his endocrine disorder change his life and destiny?

Napoleon was the second son of an impoverished Corsican aristocrat. He devoted much effort and time to his studies and became an authority on the mobile use of artillery. His rise in the army was fortuitous and rapid; at the age of twenty-seven he was appointed to command the army for the invasion of Italy. About this time he became enamored of Josephine, a beautiful Creole, widow of the Viscount de Beauharnais. He discarded his mistress Desirée, for whom he had great affection, to marry a woman who could advance his goals.

Josephine's morals were none too strict. She was a vivacious woman, a great charmer who was living at this time by her wits. Bonaparte, six years her junior, was a young tyro who had led a somewhat chaste and Spartan life. His chastity may have been due more to impecunious circumstances than a desire for celibacy. Although he made his sexual debut with a young prostitute in Lyons at the age of twenty-one, his biographers report that at eleven he was initiated into the mysteries of sex by a young woman who lived at the same pension in Ajaccio. Also, when he was twelve he was intimate with his cousin, Leonore. Despite so precocious a start, he nonetheless proved an innocent babe in the hands of Josephine. If the preacher of *Ecclesiastes* was less than chivalrous when he taught 'of woman came the beginning of sin, and through her therefore we all die', I do not believe that I am being vindictive in saying that one woman, Josephine de Beauharnais, indirectly contributed as much to Napoleon's downfall as did the might of his political and military enemies.

Napoleon's marriage to Josephine unloosed his bridled passions; their conjugal existence was sensuous, ardent, exciting. His frequent absences served only to heighten his desire for her. With the passage of time, however, her failure to conceive brought on misgivings as to his manhood. Unfortunately, he confused virility with fertility. While occupied in Egypt, he set out to prove himself. He had an adventure with a Madame Foures and was prepared to marry her if only she could become pregnant. Her inability to satisfy his yearning for fatherhood convinced him further of her sterility. Moreover, when he learned that another mistress, Eleonore Denuelle de la Plaigne, was with child, he refused to acknowledge paternity of the infant. Some years later his doubts were assuaged as the child grew to resemble him. During his absence from France he continued to have many affairs while Josephine, neglected, took her pleasures where she found them.

Napoleon's return from his campaign in Egypt was marked by two important events: he became First Consul of France; he acquired an acute case of urethritis (*la chaude pisse*). Since he had not been with another woman for at least fifty days, he strongly suspected Josephine. His physicians tried to allay his fears by assuring him that the infection was not woman-borne but simply due to *un rhume* (a cold) of the bladder—a cystitis.

Some years later Napoleon was crowned Emperor. The coronation of Napoleon and Josephine was captured on canvas by Jacques Louis David; the painting hangs in the Louvre—a reminder of a union that started off gloriously and with great promise. But the frequent bouts of urinary distress beset him with doubts. Psychogenic loss of libido is quite common when a spouse's fidelity is suspect. His sexual vigor diminished, and there may be some truth to the retort credited to him, '*pas ce soir, Josephine*' (not tonight, Josephine). In fact, this Creole adventuress did not hesitate to spread tales that he was *bon à rien* (good for nothing). She even dared to compare him to Crescentini, a then famous singer who was a castrato, implying that each merely had the appearance of a man. An incident belying his loss of sexual ardor took place in the palace at St Cloud. A French actress named Mlle George spent the night with the Emperor. During a voluptuous orgy, he lost consciousness. Frightened, she screamed for help, rousing the palace. Josephine, learning of the emergency, donned a dressing-gown and rushed to his chambers. When Napoleon came to, he found himself surrounded by his naked mistress and his clothed wife.

His attractions for other women were deep-rooted; in 1807 he fell deeply in love with a Polish girl, Marie Walewska, with whom he had an affair for several years. In May 1810 she bore him a son.

After divorcing Josephine, he married the Archduchess Marie Louise in the hopes of strengthening his political ties with Austria. He consummated his marriage by possessing her not once but twice. She, so gratified by his prowess in the boudoir, demanded an encore. Her sexual appetite was so great that during the first three months he neglected the affairs of state, devoting his attentions wholly to Marie Louise. He became so fatigued that his physician, Corvisart, cautioned moderation. She too conceived and bore him a son. About this time, drastic changes in his health occurred; his sex life began to falter. The loss of potentia at the age of forty-two was but a signal of an incipient endocrine disorder. The striking decline in his sexual powers seemed to coincide with his diminished vigor for battle, for quick decisions, for imaginative maneuvers, ending in his retreat from Moscow, his defeat at Waterloo.

Napoleon Bonaparte was another great figure who fell victim to hemorrhoids and women. Intermittent attacks of thrombosed hemorrhoids recurred during his various campaigns in Europe. During his disastrous invasion of Russia in 1812, this condition again presented and was further aggravated by urinary distress due to an old case of *chaude pisse*. His retreat from Moscow ended in his banishment to Elba. Then in the year 1815, Napoleon escaped and with a force of one thousand landed at Cannes. Thence, he began his march on Paris to reclaim the throne. The powers, fearing a repetition of the emperor's rape of Europe, allied themselves to crush him by force of arms. Battalions of Anglo-Dutch under Wellington, and Prussian troops under Blucher were deployed throughout Belgium. Napoleon believed it was imperative to destroy them before the Austrian and Russian armies could arrive at the Rhine and threaten him from the East. At dawn, June 15th, Napoleon's '*armée du nord*' crossed the Belgian frontier. He divided his army into two wings and a reserve. Marshal Ney, in command of the left, pushed on towards Wellington, while Marshal Grouchy struck at Blucher. The French advanced, stormed and captured Charleroi, the first important city across the border. In the meantime, Blucher's defeat at Ligny on June 16th rendered Wellington's position untenable. The momentum belonged to the French and the need to press forward was critical. Unfortunately, on the morning of June 17th, Napoleon arrived in a listless torpor. He was not well and was not in the saddle as early as he otherwise would have been. Discommoded by an acute case of hemorrhoids, he had been awake most of the night, finally falling asleep in the early hours of the morning. Neither of his commanders made any serious arrangements for an advance when every minute was golden. Their indecision, in the absence of Napoleon, afforded Blucher time to detach his forces and regroup and gave Wellington time to retreat to a more favorable position. Napoleon now pressed the attack and began his pursuit of Wellington but the advantage was lost. The Anglo-Dutch forces held their ground against their onslaughts and successfully counterattacked with murderous results. Napoleon was routed. In the meantime, Grouchy successfully pushed forward against the Prussians. However, on learning of the dêbacle on his left, he felt that the campaign was lost and prepared to retreat. A division under the command of the Duc de Cambron, surrounded by the resurging Prussians, was asked to surrender. He disdainfully replied '*merde*' (its equivalent is the four-letter Anglo-Saxon word for feces. The history books of France refer to it only as 'le mot de Cambron'). In a quite similar situation during World War II, the American Commander, General McAuliffe, was asked to surrender when his forces were surrounded by the Germans in their last convulsive stand at the Battle of the Bulge. His rejoinder was apparently quite simply—'nuts'. I rather suspect his terse retort was really 'le mot de Cambron'.

Napoleon lost the battle of Waterloo. He was forced to abdicate. His wife refused to accompany him when he was banished to Elba some years following the Russian débacle, or later when he was imprisoned on St Helena. He was being trumped by Count von Neipperg. It is sad to relate that his two great loves, Josephine and Marie Louise, had both cuckolded him. He who bestrode the world like a colossus, now could not even conquer mons veneris.

A mushrooming endocrinopathy began to manifest itself in varying ways: progressive weight gain, increasing lassitude, uncontrollable somnolence, temporary loss of consciousness, headaches, visual disturbances, and genital atrophy. His troubles were further compounded by bouts of indigestion, constipation, and dysuria. Urinary difficulties and lethargy had plagued him at the siege of Moscow; an acute case of hemorrhoids, an attack of urinary distress, and somnolence contributed to his indolence and lack of initiative at Waterloo. Disease now lent its aid to fate in deciding the destinies of this prodigious man.

In my opinion, after due consideration of the protean manifestations of his maladies, Napoleon was the victim of multiple endocrine adenomas (polyglandular disease). Pituitary gland failure provoked signs and symptoms of hypothyroidism (lethargy, slow pulse, chilly extremities, constipation), hypoglycemia (loss of consciousness), and hypogonadism (loss of potentia, diminishing sexual hair, atrophy of the genitals). The disorder burgeoned slowly over the years, and when he died at the age of fifty-two he had a fully blossoming Zollinger–Ellison syndrome. What is the basis for such a diagnosis? Autopsy finding revealed merely a large gastric ulcer and urinary calculi. Although there was malignant transformation of the ulcer, no metastases were found. Stigmata of endocrine disease were noted. The Zollinger–Ellison syndrome is characterized by an intractable and massive peptic ulcer in association with a parathyroid and/or pancreatic adenoma. Tumors of other endocrine glands, particularly of the pituitary, may be present. Unfortunately, the autopsy was not very thorough and the brain was not examined.

Speculation as to the cause of Napoleon's death is considerable, but on one thing there is a consensus: the gradual loss of masculinity during his last years. All who wrote about him from personal observation are in agreement that he appeared less than virile. A young Irishman, a member of the crew aboard the *Bellerophon* (the ship which carried Napoleon to English waters after his surrender in July 1815), wrote home about their most distinguished passenger: 'Buonaparte is a fine looking man, inclined to corpulency; . . . complexion French yellow, . . . big belly, . . . small white hands, and shows a good leg'.

Six years later Napoleon was dead and an autopsy was performed by Dr Antonmarchi, in the presence of several English physicians. He recorded the height as 5 feet 2 inches, the body still covered thickly with a superficial layer of fat, the hips wide, the shoulders narrow. The body had feminine characteristics; his skin was white and delicate; his hands and feet were extremely small; his reproductive organs were atrophic. One of the English physicians, witness to the autopsy, described the body as effeminate, with hardly any body hair; his pubis strongly resembled that of a woman, and his penis and testicles were very small. Another observed that 'his type of plumpness was not masculine; he had beautiful arms, rounded breasts, white soft skin, no hair, and a chest that many a woman would envy'.

The French felt that the British, as well as Antonmarchi, were prejudicial and purposeful in trying to demean the great Emperor. However, the young Irishman aboard the *Bellerophon* was in awe of Napoleon and most likely unbiased. He made two keen observations: 'inclined to corpulency and complexion French yellow'. As an endocrinologist, I can assuredly say that these two characteristics are frequently seen in eunuchoidism, particularly the lemon-like tint of the skin. Perhaps Josephine intuitively and with prophetic vision recognized Napoleon's eunuchoidal qualities when she scornfully compared him to a castrato.

The gossip and charges that Napoleon had a veritable harem during his exile to Elba and that he had many affairs while imprisoned at St Helena were founded on hearsay and malevolence. The reports by the physicians in attendance and the autopsy findings would indicate that his sexual capacity had long been defunct. The rumors about his relations with the wife of his loyal and trusted military aide, de Montholon, were in all probability mischievous mouthings. Madame de Montholon visited him often, but she was a consoling friend rather than a mistress.

At St Helena, Napoleon reached the stage when the memory of past performance becomes vivid and many a feat is retold. His trysts with Desirée, his liaison with the beautiful Polish girl, the intimacies of Marie Louise, the exciting love duels with Josephine were vicariously relived. When questioned about his mistresses, Napoleon admitted to seven, saying that was '*beaucoup trop*' (too many). He was a sensuous and sensitive man and had a flair for the poetic phrase, as shown in a letter he wrote to Josephine, passionately recalling her breasts and pubis—'*le petit sein blanc . . . la petite forêt noire*' (little white breast . . . little black forest).

Chapter 4

Peccadillos
of the
Founding Fathers

Thomas Jefferson
and Benjamin Franklin

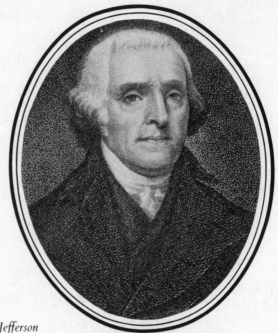

Thomas Jefferson

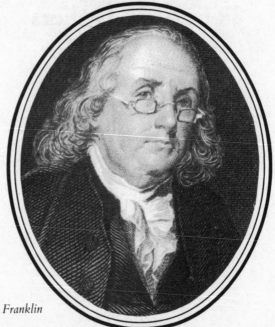

Benjamin Franklin

Thomas Jefferson

The private lives of the Founding Fathers of America have been subjected to considerable scrutiny. George Washington lusted in his heart after Sally Fairfax, but with admirable restraint let it go no further; John Adams led a life without blemish, while James Madison tarnished his by a romance with a teenage girl. The secret love-life of Thomas Jefferson and the none-too-secret one of Benjamin Franklin are sufficiently tantalizing.

Thomas Jefferson, third President of the United States, is generally regarded as a philosopher-statesman without peer. The versatility and virtuosity of this man cover the whole span of intellectual endeavor. Astronomy, chemistry, geology, botany, agronomy, and ethnology were fields well known to him. He was an educator, scientist, inventor, architect, lawyer, but something more—an arcane lover. He had a failing for the forbidden. Not generally known is the fact that Jefferson—canonized as a Founding Father without blemish in his public or private life—was indeed a passionate, guilt-ridden, secretive man whose sensual escapades have been glossed over by generations of sanctifying historians. In our own time, we have been made aware of the peccadillos of Presidents Harding, Roosevelt, and Kennedy—but to believe that Jefferson engaged in liaisons with several women seems unthinkable, almost sacrilegious.

Thomas Jefferson was a humane and rational man, whose imperfections do not diminish the achievements for which he is best remembered. His love-life was not really a sordid one; his ambiguous position regarding slavery was colored by his dalliance with a mulatto slave girl. Perhaps the reader will understand how Jefferson might write to George Washington, 'Come to Monticello, I have two virgin slave girls for you'. Whether or not this invitation was extended in jest, this roguery reveals Jefferson's 'other' side. A medical colleague, whose veracity I have no reason to doubt, claims that he read such a letter which supposedly lies buried in the Archives of the University of Virginia. As intimacies in the life of the man who drafted the Declaration of Independence are unveiled, an extraordinary and ambivalent figure appears.

Undoubtedly some will feel outraged at such innuendo and view it as a canard which should be rejected by all who love and respect the memory of a most remarkable American. But the student of human behavior must bare the facts—the truth will out! Moreover, nobody likes to think about the Founding Fathers of our country in any way that reduces them to the level of ordinary mortals. Americans hold high their heroes of bygone days and will not suffer their images to be tarnished. Indeed, Jefferson was one of the great philosophers of the eighteenth century; a kindly man who believed passionately in the worth of ordinary people and in their right and ability to govern themselves. Jefferson was probably neither saint nor sinner, but a human being subject to the same desires, temptations and conceits common to the men of his genre.

Jefferson was married to Martha Wayles, the daughter of a socially prominent, wealthy plantation owner. He described their union as ten years of unchequered happiness, and when widowed at thirty-nine, took the loss so deeply to heart that he was inconsolable for many months. Sometime thereafter he was appointed Minister Plenipotentiary to negotiate the peace in Paris. He found much to admire in France but was quite lonely, and, at times, given to bouts of melancholy. Then he was introduced into society by his friend LaFayette, and was delighted by the French women, their femininity, manners, cultivated conversation, and interest in art and music. He developed a new life-style with a trace of gallantry that endeared him to many prominent ladies of the land. Nonetheless, it was an Englishwoman who finally caught his fancy. He met Maria Cosway—the wife of Richard Cosway, a popular painter of miniatures—at a dinner party. He saw her frequently, found her irresistible, and fell madly in love. After she returned to England, he wrote her letters that were, according to historian Fawn Brodie, 'missives of such ineffable tenderness that they constitute the most remarkable collection of love letters in the history of the American Presidency'. He pleaded in one, 'If your letters are long . . . they will be short to me. Only let them be brimful of affection'. Actually, her letters were quite brief. The few weeks' flirtation with the longlimbed Virginian was for her merely an amorous interlude, and soon Jefferson was again lonely and bereft. He wrote to her, 'I am born to lose everything I love'.

During his sojourn in Paris, Jefferson sent for his little daughter, Polly. With her came Sally Hemings, a pretty mulatto nurse of fourteen. She was described as 'very handsome'and 'mighty near white'. Jefferson probably found her so. Several months after their arrival home two years later, Sally Hemings gave birth to a child. Current gossip named Jefferson as the father.

Although Jefferson may have been opposed intellectually to miscegenation, his father-in-law, John Wayles, and his mentor, George White, as well as many plantation owners, had slave concubines. This had become a custom not uncommon among the landed gentry of Virginia and the South in general.

Some thirteen years after Jefferson's return from France, he became President of the United States. James T. Callendar, coeditor of the *Richmond Recorder*, was one of many political enemies who hoped to destroy him by attacking his private life. On September 2 1802, he published: 'It is well known that the man, whom it delighted the people to honor, keeps, and for many years has kept, as his concubine, one of his slaves. Her name is Sally. The name of her oldest is Tom. His features are said to bear a striking though sable resemblance to the President himself'. Callendar was determined to further embarrass the President by resurrecting an old rumor that, before his own marriage, Jefferson had tried to seduce Betsy Walker, the wife of one of his best friends. Jefferson admitted privately, in a now-famous letter, 'When young and single, I offered love to a handsome lady; I acknowledge its incorrectness'. But he never admitted that Sally Hemings was his slave-mistress or that he had fathered any of her several children. One fact, however, was brought out in an account written by the editor of the *Frederick-Town Herald*: Sally, unlike the other slaves, had a room to herself in the big house where she performed her duties as seamstress. But there was a plausible reason for this preferential treatment, since Sally, the beautiful quadroon, was in fact a half-sister to Jefferson's deceased wife. John Wayles, after the death of his third wife, had turned to Elizabeth Hemings—a slave on his plantation who was the daughter of an English sea captain and an African slave woman. Elizabeth bore Wayles six children; the youngest was Sally. After Wayles died, the children came to Monticello as part of Martha Wayles' inheritance.

Many charges were heaped upon President Jefferson in the venomous Federalist press, and the abuses he took concerning his private life have never been fully told. Despite the savagery of the attacks, including numerous bawdy ballads—one of them written by John Quincy Adams—he kept Sally and her children at Monticello. Whether or not they were his children, Jefferson refused to be intimidated; and he paid dearly for keeping them.

He was also criticized for the influence of his five-year sojourn in France on his manners, morals, and political philosophy. He often regaled his colleagues with stories of the private lives of European diplomats. Senator Maclay, of Pennsylvania, expressed shock at what he considered such lax talk about women, and felt that Jefferson 'had been long enough abroad to catch the tone of European folly'.

Somehow, he remained a singularly sweet-tempered man, and his kindness of heart rose above the bitterness that raged about him. All his life he cultivated a serene, civilized good humor; and perhaps that is how he bore with relative equanimity the flood of coarse and malignant abuse of his motives, morals, religion, personal honesty and decency. In 1805, the President wrote a letter to his Attorney General, Levi Lincoln, and his Secretary of State, Robert Smith, in an attempt to extricate himself from the web of those many allegations. Mysteriously, these letters—which could prove his innocence or guilt—have disappeared.

With the passage of time, it has generally been conceded that Thomas Jefferson was probably the greatest of all our Presidents. Yet he never enriched himself at the public trough; and no one was more generous than he was with his money and time in the service of his nation, which he helped to found and mold. One of his great accomplishments was the Statute of Virginia for Religious Freedom, which he authored. It served as the model that enabled men of all faiths to seek public office in these United States. Uriah

Levy, a man belonging to the Jewish faith, was so moved by this act of tolerance that he commissioned the most famous sculptor of the day, Pierre D'Angers of France, to do a massive bronze of Jefferson. His gift was accepted by Congress and the statue presently stands to the right of George Washington in the Capitol Rotunda.

Upon completion of his second term as President, Jefferson found himself hopelessly in debt. In order to pay off his creditors, he had no other choice but to sell his great library and all but 409 acres of his 10,000 acre estate. Although he died without a cent to his name, he left a priceless legacy to mankind: 'All men are created equal . . . endowed with certain inalienable rights . . . life, liberty, and the pursuit of happiness'.

However, the concepts of equality expressed in this great document did not extend to Jefferson's private life. His mulatto concubine was never accorded a 'born equal' status—she was denied her inalienable rights and merely served as an outlet for his androgenic drives, only in accordance with his pursuit of happiness. And as Jefferson grew in stature, this confluence of forces compelled him to defy convention and restraint as he fought for his inalienable right to sexual freedom.

Benjamin Franklin

Two hundred years ago, seventy-year-old Benjamin Franklin was appointed to the committee responsible for framing the Declaration of Independence. Wise and full of years, he struck the words 'sacred and undeniable' from Jefferson's original draft, 'We hold these truths to be sacred and undeniable, that all men are created equal', and he substituted 'self-evident'. Herein lies the measure of the most resourceful of the Founding Fathers—a man who opted, at all times, for simplicity and forthrightness—in speech, in dress, and in action. The magnitude of his accomplishments and diversity of his interests make it difficult to distill the essence of his personality and obtain a unified portrait of the man who passed into American legend well before his death at the age of eighty-four.

How could a poor Boston boy, the youngest son of a family of seventeen, who had but two years of schooling, grow to such eminence? At twelve he was apprenticed to his older brother, who had a printing shop, and a few years later, he moved to Philadelphia, where he began his life-long career in printing and publishing. He prepared himself by reading as many books and pamphlets as he could obtain, from the Bible to the works of Shakespeare. As a young man he authored the highly popular and financially successful *Poor Richard's Almanac*. He taught himself the basic principles of algebra, geometry, grammar, logic, and the physical and natural sciences, partially mastered French, Italian, Spanish and Latin, and learned to play several musical instruments. He made of himself one of the most educated men of his time. As his business ventures flourished, he began to devote more and more of his energy and talent to the public good. He established the world's first subscription library, organized the city's Fire Department, improved the postal service, raised money to build a community hospital, organized the American Philosophical Society, helped found the academy that eventually grew into the University of Pennsylvania, and formulated plans for a medical school. He was repeatedly elected or appointed to a number of political posts and was Pennsylvania's representative to the First Continental Congress.

As a scientist and inventor, he showed the world that lightning was actually electricity and that farming could be improved by adding lime to the soil. He invented bifocal glasses, the lightning rod, the Franklin stove, and a musical instrument (the harmonica). His scientific achievements earned him membership of the Royal Society of London and the Society's Copley Medal, membership of the French Academy of Science, and honorary degrees from Harvard and Oxford.

As a statesman and diplomat, he represented Pennsylvania and several of the other colonies in Great Britain for the greater part of eighteen years (1757–1775), and then was appointed minister to France, a post he held from 1776 to 1785. No other American, except possibly Thomas Jefferson, did so many things so well. He was truly America's first Renaissance man.

Franklin had his own code of morality and bothered little about prevailing conventions. He was an unpretentious man who scorned pomposity and abhorred self-righteousness and hypocrisy. Few things were sacred to him, including formalized religion, for he was a free-thinker. All his life, he could not regulate his sexual impulses and lusted after women hungrily, secretly, and briefly. Franklin confessed 'that hard to be governed passion of youth hurried me frequently into intrigues with low women—a continual risk to my health by a distemper which by great luck I escaped . . .'. At twenty-four, he took Deborah Reed to wife without benefit of clergy and surprised her by bringing along the first of his illegitimate offspring. Although he fell deeply in love at the age of forty-eight with Miss Catherine Ray, a young, beautiful, intelligent Boston lady, and although he had a long 'platonic' relationship with the charming Mrs Margaret Stephenson, his landlady in London, he never revealed any intimate sexual contacts he may have had with them or the many ladies he cultivated at home and abroad. He did admit making numerous improper advances, but his attitude toward womankind and sex was genteel, respectful, appreciative, and discreet. Nevertheless, the image persists that he warmed more beds in Philadelphia than most people realized.

Franklin was one of the first American writers to exploit sex in his colorful stories and fables. His Rabelaisian humor is evident in a letter he wrote in answer to a fictitious inquiry, 'On the Choice of a Mistress'. Marriage he wrote, 'is the most natural state of man but . . .', he admonished, 'if you cannot take this counsel and persist in thinking a commerce with the sex inevitable, then . . . in all your amours you should prefer old women to young ones'. Some of the reasons he offered were:

because the sin is less; the debauching of a virgin may be her ruin and make her life unhappy; because the compunction is less; the having made a young girl miserable may give you frequent and bitter reflection, none of which can attend making an old woman happy; and lastly, they are grateful! . . : But still I advise you to marry directly.

By interjecting a salacious flavour into the articles published in his newspaper, *The Pennsylvania Gazette*, he increased its circulation and assured its success.

Franklin believed that most goals were attainable through persistence, effort, imagination, and, if necessary, caprice. It was just such a man who was needed to find help and support for the newly founded nation. The colonists desperately needed an ally that would furnish arms and money; otherwise, the rebellion would surely fail. Soon after completing his stint on the committee to prepare the Declaration of Independence, Franklin was chosen to present the cause of the rebelling colonists to England's avowed enemy, France. During his first year in Paris, he could no nothing to cajole Louis XVI to come to the aid of America. But with inordinate diplomatic skill as well as considerable maneuvering—and not without some connivance—he finally extracted an alliance from France, which meant all-out assistance to the beleaguered colonists and a war with England. Ultimately the British were forced to make peace with their former colonies. The peace Treaty was signed in 1783, a personal victory for the now seventy-seven-year-old diplomat.

The Americans won an impossible war with the aid of the French through the Treaty of Alliance, which Franklin had secured from the King of France. How was he able to accomplish this feat? He charmed. He persevered. He endeared himself, both to the aristocracy and the common people. His reputation as a *bon vivant*, a wit, a philosopher, and a scientist preceded him. His book on electricity was revolutionary and startling, and his almanac was quite popular because of its humorous aphorisms. He was a lovable old eccentric and was lionized by the society matrons of Paris. He courted several of them actively, frequently using them to influence political leaders on behalf of the Americans.

During his nine-year sojourn in France, from the ages of seventy to seventy-nine, he may have made many mistakes and his record was marred by some inexcusable failures, but none occurred in his relationship with women. He was adored by the highest ladies of the court and by the lowest chambermaids. Of the Founding

Fathers, George Washington and Thomas Jefferson had great admiration for him; John Adams had little and once sarcastically remarked, 'Franklin, at the age of seventy-odd, had neither lost his love of beauty nor his taste for it'. In his old age, Franklin's pursuit of the ladies was courtly but often naughty. He made many amorous advances which usually came to naught. He was an undaunted optimist but it seems that his desire outdistanced his performance. He apparently believed this his gout was worsened by the reduction in sexual pleasures, for with gay badinage he wrote to one of his favorites, Madame Brillon de Jouy, 'When I was a young man and enjoyed more favors from sex than at present, I never had the gout. If the ladies of Passy had more Christian charity which I have so often recommended to you, in vain, I would not have the gout now'.

At seventy-nine, America's first ambassador to France returned triumphantly to the United States. His place in Paris was taken by Thomas Jefferson who said, 'I am not replacing Franklin—no one could do that. I am only his successor'. Franklin the elder statesman, although in constant pain with gout, spent his time quietly reading, writing, and working in his laboratory. At eighty-one, he was once again called upon, this time to draft a new constitution for the newly formed United States of America, and in September 1787, the new constitution was signed. Franklin was the only one of the Founding Fathers whose name appears on all four documents that turned the British Colonies into an independent nation. His signature is on the Declaration of Independence, the treaty of alliance with France, the treaty of peace with England, and the Constitution of the United States.

Franklin died three years later at the age of eighty-four. He hoped that after his death people would say of him, 'He lived usefully', rather than, 'he died rich'. Indeed, he did not die rich, but the heritage he left is immeasurable. Society is often the beneficiary of untold wealth bequeathed to it by men considered long past their prime. Longfellow in his 'Morituri Salutamus' saluted men of his genre:

Ah, nothing is too late
Till the tired heart shall cease to palpitate . . .
Chaucer at Woodstock with the nightingales
At sixty wrote The Canterbury Tales,
Goethe at Weimar, toiling to the last,
Completed Faust when eighty years past . . .
For age is opportunity no less
Than youth itself, though in another dress . . .

Franklin's life, especially the last twenty-five years, was rich, varied, productive, and legendary. His world revolved around a host of interests—'from cabbages to kings'.

Chapter 5

 # Distorted passions

*Adolph Hitler
and Reichsmarshal
Hermann Goering*

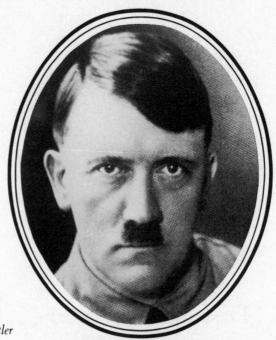

Adolf Hitler

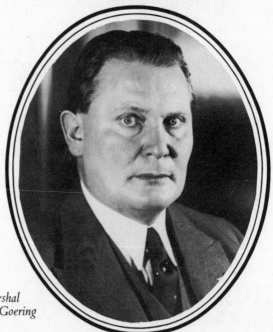

*Reichsmarshal
Hermann Goering*

Adolph Hitler

The sex life of Adolf Hitler has been the subject of endless and so far inconclusive speculation. Historians and students of human behavior should rightly be concerned with the sexual antics of this man who stands condemned as the vilest architect of mass murder in the memory of man. There is a lesson to be learned.

Hitler's early years were marked by a disturbed parent–child upbringing. At the age of twelve, he was reprimanded by school authorities for molesting a little girl. Several years later, his application for art school was turned down. Frustrated and unhappy in his home town of Linz, he left for Vienna, where he remained for more than four years. There he lived in squalor and abject poverty, working at odd jobs if and when the spirit moved him. This ne'er-do-well lived in public flophouses and stayed alive by begging in the streets, eating at free soup-kitchens, and by selling hand-painted postcards. He was a shiftless and angry young man who wallowed in the filth of his surroundings while associating with the dregs of humanity. How this unschooled, undisciplined, asocial, nondescript person could mesmerize and seduce a highly civilized nation into blind allegiance remains a mystery. His psychosexual problems remained bottled up in him, seeking release, and he probably felt cheated in that he had only one testicle. When poor and powerless, he thirsted for power; when alone, alienated, and tortured, he had a compulsion to torture others. Having debased himself, he wanted to debase the human race. Because of him forty million people died. The elements of depravity, of a twisted and sick mind, should have been detected long before he became 'der Fuehrer'—the supreme overlord of Germany.

The innate irresponsibility, the savageness of this demonic genius was blazingly brought into view when he ordered his retreating forces to destroy the most beautiful city in the world. What occupied his thoughts most at that very moment was the question—'Is Paris burning?' He once stated, 'We shall not capitulate—no never. We may be destroyed, but if we are, we shall drag a world with us—a world in flames'. None will deny that he was a sadist of the first order. The furnaces of Buchenwald, the gas chambers of Auschwitz stand as mute memorials to the six million Jews and five million other non-combatants and political prisoners who died so ignominiously. A universal symbol of sadism is the whip, and like the notorious bully of the Nazi Party, Julius Streicher, Hitler too was fond of strutting with his rawhide bull-whip in his hand. Being a sadist was but one side of the coin. That he was also a masochist was known only to a few. A study of his sexual exploits, or lack of them, can be pieced together from the facts at hand, from hearsay, and from psychological interpretations of his relationships with males and females.

What is the evidence for his unnatural sexual conduct? Hitler had a visual–oral–anal fixation that manifested itself in a variety of ways.

Masochistic Perversion
In her description of sexual experiences with Hitler, his niece, Geli Raubal, stressed that it was of utmost importance to him that she squat over his face in such a way that he could see everything. How often he practised this extreme form of masochistic degradation with Geli will never be known for she committed suicide after a dalliance of two years.

He practised less degrading activities when the relationship was frivolous or less secure. The actress, Rene Mueller, much troubled after spending a night with Hitler, expiated her sin by confessing to Ziessler, her director. According to his report, it appears that instead of bedding down, Hitler fell to the floor and begged her to kick him. She demurred, but he pleaded with her until she finally acceded to his wishes. As she continued to kick him, he became more and more excited. Rene Mueller committed suicide shortly after this experience.

Hitler had relatively few affairs with women. He was afraid that if an intimate relationship did develop and warm feelings of affection asserted themselves, the compulsion to degrade himself would become too strong. His struggle for control of this urge was ever uppermost. The situation was so enervating and so frustrating that, unknowingly, he compensated for this inner turmoil by frequent and uncontrollable 'rages'. It is indeed odd that of the few women who were intimate with Hitler, almost all attempted or succeeded in committing suicide. Those who attempted to kill themselves include Unity Mitford, Martha Dodd, Suzi Liptauer, Marie Reiter and Inge Ley. Eva Braun tried twice to take her own life. She who loved him selflessly for years and had proven her obedience by complying with his unusual sexual demands, finally took potassium cyanide immediately after Hitler's suicide.

Was Hitler a Homosexual?
Many writers and informants have commented on Hitler's feminine characteristics. Putzi Hanfstaengl, a confidant of Hitler during his early days in Bavaria said, 'he was incapable of intercourse'. A specimen of Hitler's handwriting was shown to the famous psychiatrist, Dr Jung, who proclaimed that the handwriting was typically feminine. Hitler's hands were small and female-like. His choice of art as a profession (painting postcards) may be interpreted as a manifestation of basic feminine identification. Many commented on his gait as being ladylike. For years Hitler was suspected of being a homosexual, although there is no reliable evidence that he actually engaged in a relationship of this kind. The most that can be said is that circumstantial evidence (see below) would indict him if guilt by association and hearsay were permissible evidence.

(1) After Hitler became prominent in Munich politics, a photographer, Heinrich Hoffman, became quite friendly with him. After Hoffman's wife died, his house became a rendezvous for homosexuals of both sexes. Hitler must have committed some kind of sexual indiscretion with Hoffman's daughter, Henny, which enraged her father. Hitler bought Hoffman's silence by granting him exclusive rights as the official 'Party' photographer, and arranged for Henny to marry Baldur von Sirach, the leader of the Nazi youth movement, who was reputed to be a homosexual.

(2) Hermann Rauschning, author of several articles on Hitler, reported that he met two boys who claimed that they were Hitler's

homosexual partners.

(3) Foerster, the Danzig gauleiter, a known homosexual, was intimate enough to be on a 'first name' basis with Hitler. He implied that the Reichsfuehrer was impotent as far as heterosexual relations were concerned.

(4) Hitler permitted several notorious homosexuals in his 'Nazi cabinet'. Roehm was brazen about it, while Hess was known as 'Fraulein Anna'. His second chief in command, Hermann Goering, with his transvestite tendencies, is a study in himself. The early Nazi party certainly contained many members with sexual aberrations. Captain von Mueke succinctly stated, 'It is a pigsty' as his reason for resigning from the Party.

(5) For years, Hitler chose to live with the dregs of society in a Vienna flophouse known to be inhabited by many homosexuals. It is probably for this reason he was listed on the Vienna police records as a 'sexual pervert'—an entry made solely on suspicions.

(6) Otto Strasser reported that Hitler's personal bodyguards were almost always a hundred per cent homosexual, and that Hitler derived pleasure from looking at men's bodies and associating with homosexuals.

Preoccupation with Feces and the Buttocks
In 'Mein Kampf', Hitler repeatedly referred to the miserable years he spent in Vienna as a time of extreme hardship, but he never really tried to improve his lot. He seemed to take pleasure in his humiliation, for his attitude was . . . 'I enjoy nothing more than to lie around while the world defecates on me'. Psychoanalyst Langer, in his remarkable book, *The Mind of Adolf Hitler*, explains Hitler's preoccupation with filth and excreta:

> He abandoned the genital level of libidinal development and became impotent as far as heterosexual relations were concerned. . . . When a regression of this kind takes place, the sexual instinct usually becomes diffuse, and many organs that have yielded some sexual stimulation in the past become permanently invested with sexual significance. The eyes, for example,

may become a substitute sexual organ and seeing then takes on a sexual significance.

It was known that Hitler delighted in observing striptease and nude dancing. He frequently invited such entertainers to perform in private, and he often invited girls to Berchtesgaden for the purpose of exhibiting their bodies. On his walls were countless pictures of obscene nudes, and he was especially delighted with a collection of pornographic pictures which Hoffman had compiled for him. In addition to the eyes, the anal region became highly sexualized with both feces and buttocks as sexual objects. The historian, Robert G. L. Waite, wrote that while Hitler saw himself as a veritable Messiah of his people, he also referred to himself as a *'scheisskerl'* (shithead).

In *The Life and Death of Adolf Hitler* by Robert Payne, the author makes the statement that Hitler chose the code names of his military offenses carefully, and these were frequently meaningful. He chose 'Barbarossa' for his attack and invasion of Russia. The original Barbarossa (Redbeard) was the German Emperor Frederick I (1123–1190). The great conqueror brought Bohemia, Hungary and Poland under his sway, but he could not forget the ignominy of defeat by a small body of Milanese pikemen at Legarno. He was determined to revenge this wound to his ego by contemptuously ordering the people of Milan 'to remove with their teeth a fig which had become lodged in the anus of his mule'. So, too, Hitler's aim was not merely to conquer the Russians but also to make them, figuratively speaking, eat *dreck* (filth, excreta). Perhaps that is why he named his campaign 'Barbarossa'—Hitler was a spiteful man and had contempt for the human race. Though he had a Messiah complex, he seems actually to have been the devil incarnate. In Christian iconography it is not unusual to encounter a parallelism between the devil and sexuality, and also between the devil and the anus. Martin Luther, the leader of the Reformation, was quite visionary when he ascribed to the devil the saying . . . 'I am the turd that is ready and the world is the wide open anus'. *Nascimur inter feces et urinam* (we are born between feces and urine)—but

Adolph Hitler never strayed too far from the feces and urine.

Reichsmarshal Hermann Goering

September 1 1939, was a memorable day for Reichsmarshal Hermann Goering. He gloried in the fact that his regenerated Luftwaffe was in combat over Warsaw—the invasion of Poland had begun. A few days later he had further reason to rejoice. He stood to inherit a considerable estate, for Lily Epenstein, his surrogate mother, had died suddenly. She had been on a secret mission to America and had hurriedly returned just before hostilities broke out. Hermann Goering, bastard son of the rich Hermann Epenstein, had risen high in the National Socialist hierarchy and the widowed Mrs Epenstein, distrustful of the Nazis, wisely sought Goering's protection; he, in turn, used her position and wealth to further his ambitions and designs.

What is the Goering story? What kind of man was he? How did his psychophysical disorder color his life pattern? What of his parentage?

In the town of Metz, a Judge Goering was physically attracted to and infatuated with a pretty flower girl and sometime waitress, whom he married. The alliance was frowned upon by his peers and he faced banishment to one of the colonies or mandatory resignation from his judgeship. He chose to accept a post in Walfisch Bay in West Africa. There his wife bore him two children, both girls. After a few years, the Goerings were on a trip back to Europe. Aboard the ship was a Mr Hermann Epenstein, a wealthy bachelor who was in the habit of appropriating the things that pleased him. He met Mrs Goering, liked what he saw, and invited the Goering family to live with him in his beautiful castle-fortress. There, the now retired judge, a confirmed wine-bibber, drank himself slowly out of life, for Epenstein kept an excellent wine cellar. The platonic friendship of Mr Epenstein and Mrs Goering blossomed and she soon found herself with child. A son was born and named Hermann. Shortly thereafter, the intemperate judge died. Some months after his death, a second son was born to Mrs Goering; this one was christened Albert. Hermann Epenstein provided an education for the two boys and a dowry for Mrs Goering's two daughters, but never considered marriage to her. Epenstein fell ill during the First World War, and the nurse who diligently watched over him and broke him of his morphine addiction ultimately became his wife, much to the chagrin of Mrs Goering. Lily Epenstein was a charming and reasonable lady and she helped breach the rift that her marriage created—particularly with Hermann Goering, now that he had become a powerful figure in the Nazi party.

In 1934, Hermann Epenstein, now eighty-four years of age, persuaded Albert to visit his brother in Berlin. Albert had shown disdain for Hermann, calling him a 'political impersonator'. However, he fulfilled his father's wish and was received by Hermann, who was gowned in purple robes, sitting on some kind of throne, flanked by a lion on one side and a Great Dane on the other. Amused by this sight, Albert inquired, 'Hermann, are you so courageous, or are you afraid?' The brothers, though philosophically and politically poles apart, made peace with each other, much to their father's satisfaction. Epenstein died that same year and willed that his property be divided between his two illegitimate sons after his wife's demise. Perhaps then the death of Lily Epenstein, so soon after her return from America, takes on new meaning.

What circumstances fashioned Goering's life? One thing is certain, his successes on the politico-military front were in contrast to the frustrations and failures in his love-life. As a boy, he grew up in the lap of luxury, having all the amenities with which the rich provide their children. He lived in a castle, and in his reveries he envisioned the medieval family, the Knights of Epenstein, as his distant progenitors. He became an outrageously flamboyant individualist, whose life was destined to be a strange mixture of gaiety, excitement, and vanity. He was given to wine and food, women and drugs, and there were elements of the exhibitionist and transvestite in him.

When Hermann Goering, now in the uniform of the army, un-expectedly developed arthritis in 1914, at the age of twenty-one he thought his career was at an end. Yet he overcame his infirmity and was soon training as a pilot in the fledgling air force. He had great ability and qualities of leadership, and in 1917 was given a command of his own, Jasta 27. He participated in many campaigns and personally downed several enemy planes. In July 1918, Oberleut-nant Hermann Goering was appointed commander of the most prestigious air wing, named after the great German ace Von Richt-hofen. However, within three months German resistance col-lapsed and the Armistice was signed on November 11 1918. Goering was instructed to lead his squadron to Aschaffenburg for the purpose of surrendering the aircraft to a French commission. As a final act of defiance, he admonished his pilots to deliberately land the planes in such a manner as to wreck them. Thus, the Impe-rial German Air Force—*im kreig geboren, im kreig gestorben* (born in war, died in war)—brought its valiant history to a close. The disil-lusioned Goering was contemptuous of his Fatherland in defeat. He accepted a job as an aircraft salesman in Scandinavia, where he married the Countess Rosen and enjoyed a gay and luxurious life in Sweden. The marriage was not a happy one and the Countess sued for divorce. Some time before the divorce could take place, she died. One might ask, 'Of natural causes?' After the death of the Countess, Goering ended his self-imposed exile by returning to Munich, where he enrolled at the University in 1921.

One evening he listened to an incongruous, nondescript rabble-rouser with an odd moustache haranguing a crowd, demanding vengeance and restoration of the glory that once was Germany's. The stirring violence of the man attracted him and he sought a meeting. Adolph Hitler perceived that the much-decorated former leader of the Von Richthofen Squadron would be a valuable asset to the German Workers Party. His social standing and remarkable war record would give 'class' to an organization still composed mostly of the uneducated working people. Hitler offered Goering command of the infamous strong-arm goon squads, known as the brown-shirted stormtroopers. It was the experience for which Goering longed—one that promised authority, showmanship, glamor, and a chance to vent a latent sadistic streak. He took the first step on the long road that would eventually lead him to the depths of degradation and to suicide in a lonely prison cell.

Goering became the second most important man in the Third Reich. The fat, bemedaled Reichsmarshal enjoyed a popularity among the masses second only to Hitler's, but for opposite reasons. Where Hitler was distant, legendary, nebulous, and an enigma as a human being, Goering was a salty, earthy, lusty man of flesh and blood. The Germans admired him because he had faults and strengths; he had a child's love for uniforms and medals; he had a passion for good food and much drink. He loved medieval pomp, marble halls, colorful costumes, and the fantastic. He built a magnificent palace outside of Berlin, and there had constructed a majestic mausoleum where he had the body of his late wife, Countess Rosen, brought from Sweden and laid to rest. He presented the façade of a jolly fat man, but behind this exterior there was another Goering—he who had organized the mass executions on the 'night of the long knives', and took more than a casual interest in the new policy for the complete extermination of the Jews. Behind the man of mirth there lurked a fat, capon-like male who lusted for sexual feats and exploits with a never-ending search for gratification that remained beyond his grasp. The author of *Ecclesiastes* understood full well the frustrations and inner turmoil experienced by the physical and psychological eunuch when he employed the simile 'Like a eunuch's craving to ravish a girl' (20:4). Nonetheless, Goering became enamoured of a second-rate actress, Emi Sonneman, whom he married on April 10 1935—resplendent in the uniform of a *General der Flieger*. The wedding was so outlandishly lavish that it earned the scorn of the Minister of Propaganda, Joseph Goebbels.

Despite the tantalizing and luscious Emi Sonneman, Goering found that his sexual powers were lacking. About this time, there was a stirring in the hormonal research field for a sexual elixir. Professor Fred Koch was toiling with bull testicles in Chicago,

Butenandt was extracting oceans of urine in Gottingen, and Ruzicka was dabbling with cholesterol in Zurich. Rumor was current that Leopold Ruzicka had synthesized testosterone. This chemical agent was capable of restoring to a caponized rooster the growth of the cock's comb and wattles, the capacity to crow, and the drive to chase hens. Ruzicka and Budenandt were later awarded the Noble Prize for their contribution to science; the Nazis, however, forced Budenandt to decline it. There is a story circulating amongst endocrinologists, probably apocryphal, that Goering appealed to Ruzicka for testosterone. The scientist remonstrated that the hormone was still experimental and had not been employed in the human, and he was wary of using it until further tests could be performed. Goering, however, cajoled him into making it available to him. Ruzicka finally agreed, but insisted that Goering let him know how he fared because this was the first human trial. A message was to be sent phrased in algebraic terms if the result was fair; 'trigonometry' if good; 'calculus' if excellent. Several weeks later, a telegram arrived, 'Failed in higher mathematics, but passed Romance languages'. To maintain his front of virility, Emi Sonneman conceived and gave birth to a daughter. Through the indiscretion of the wife of a prominent professor, my informer told me that conception had taken place by artificial insemination.

When in 1943 the tides of war were turning, Goering fell into disfavor with Hitler because of his indolence and failure to exert his energies upon his immediate tasks. He was preoccupied with ransacking the art museums of Europe and amassing a fortune by buying up, for a pittance, the wealthy Jewish corporations that were forced into liquidation. Offended by Hitler's criticisms of his leadership of the Air Force, he deliberately withdrew to his summer house in Obersalzburg for a long vacation. There Albert Speers, the Minister of Armaments, went to see him. Goering was glad to receive him and came tripping down the stairway in his flowing green velvet dressing gown adorned with an oversized ruby brooch. Speers was astonished to find that Goering's fingernails were lacquered and his face obviously rouged.

On April 30 1945, Hitler committed suicide in the Bunker that housed his suite. Germany had lost the war and Goering was again to witness the willful destruction of many war planes so that they would not fall into enemy hands. The last aircraft of Goering's vaunted Luftwaffe lay scattered and grounded. At this juncture, he decided to seek out General Eisenhower in the hope of negotiating peace terms. He set out in his Mercedes, dressed in the grey-blue uniform of the Luftwaffe, with only three medals and his diamondstudded marshal's baton in his right hand. He reached the headquarters of the American thirty-sixth Division and was shown the usual courtesies. While waiting for the officer in charge to arrange for a 'man-to-man' chat with Eisenhower, he had a hot bath, changed his silk underwear, and drank champagne. General Eisenhower was furious when he learned of the friendly reception given the Reichsmarshal and immediately had him whisked away to Augsburg for interrogation. His medals and baton were confiscated and while under detention, his vast intake of drugs was reduced to eighteen pills per day. Finally, he was brought to Nuremberg to stand trial before the International Military Tribunal where he was found guilty of war crimes unique in their enormity. The sentence was death by hanging, but he cheated the hangman by taking potassium cyanide. He had prepared for suicide by successfully concealing on his person a tiny metal container with the poison.

What can be said about this man? Hermann Wilhelm Goering, the fighter pilot of the First World War, later to become Marshal of the Greater Reich, was a cunning, deceitful, and vindictive man, given to boasting and childish temper. He was blinded by vanity, he craved riches and sought a life of luxury. As an endocrinologist I see the byproduct of a disordered glandular system. The least that can be said is that Goering suffered from a pseudo-Frohlich syndrome—a disturbance marked by obesity and exceptionally small genitals; this beaming, rosy-cheeked jester laughed when he was called 'the fat man'. He was consumed with the need to prove himself—as much by the acquisition of material things as with matters sexual. He had many women, though more as a disguise than an index of performance. He was a dope addict who flaunted his craving for morphine as an undeniable right—comparable to the medieval *droit de seigneur*. He lived more ostentatiously than the richest Maharajah. He dressed in the most garish uniforms and gawdy finery; diamond rings bulged on three fingers of his small hands. His sexual inadequacy and effeminate nature shone through despite his cloak of virility (hunter, marksman, fighter-pilot, *bon vivant*, womanizer). He compensated by an odd mixture of ruthless efficiency and goodhumored devilment. Goering behaved like an adult eunuch in his fat and capon-like appearance; a change that came over him shortly after the First World War. Later, frustrated, dejected vengeful, addicted to dope and food, he could no longer sublimate his compulsion to ravish the human race. Brendan Behan, in *Borstal Boy*, mockingly recalled the rhyme about the leaders of the Third Reich:

> Hitler has only got one ball,
> Goering has two but very small,
> Himmler has something similar,
> But poor old Goebbels has no balls at all.

Chapter 6

A surfeit of sex

Casanova and Mussolini

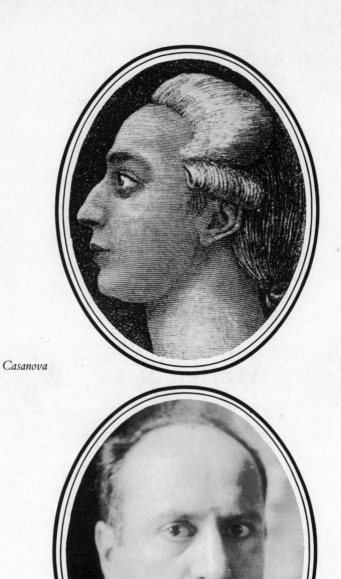

Casanova

Mussolini

Casanova

Legends of Alexander the Great, Genghis Khan, and Napoleon will endure, but the names of many other conquerors are all but forgotten. One name, that of a conqueror of a different genre, has become a byword in the language of Western man. The name—a synonym for the romantically promiscuous man—is Casanova.

Jacques Casanova was born in Venice in 1725 and died, probably a syphilitic, seventy-three years later. He lived a life full of adventure and intrigue, and made an art of seduction. He was a man of many talents: journalist, abbé, diplomat, spy, alchemist, businessman, gambler, a man of letters who wrote several books, but first and foremost, a womanizer. By his own count, he had more than a hundred love affairs and innumerable brief encounters. His *Memoirs* not only recorded his sexual exploits but were also a clever and interesting commentary of eighteenth-century manners. Another book, *Icosomerson*, recounted fantastic adventures in a fantastic world with many anticipations of modern inventions. His *History of Poland* foretold how this hapless country would be torn limb from limb by Russia and the kingdom of Prussia. In his lifetime, the prophecy came true. It happened again when Hitler connived with Stalin to sunder Poland apart—the forerunner of the Second World War.

Like biblical Cain, doomed by the Almighty to wander over the face of the earth and find no solace, Casanova was forever on the move. He found himself at one time or another in Rome, Constantinople, Paris, London, Berlin, St Petersburg, Warsaw, Madrid, and many, many other places. He never stuck to one vocation, was never rich enough, hardly ever out of debt, and always in and out of trouble. Imprisoned, expelled, scandalized, he nonetheless mingled with the famous in high society and was befriended by kings, princes and the nobility. At last, tired and spent, he retired to the Château of Duchov in Bohemia where Count Waldstein appointed him librarian.

What kind of man was Casanova? What made him run? At the age of sixteen, he was expelled from the seminary for scandalous and immoral conduct. After a few years of employment in the household of Cardinal Acquaviva, he set a course for fame and fortune. Along the way, he took the greatest pleasure in deceiving his fellowman and seducing every possible woman who attracted him. It was a compelling force that seemingly he could not control, for he risked fortune, social status, his very life—as if he could not live without the adventure. He was basically a rogue—a satyr whose breadth of conquest ranged from ten-year-old girls to seventy-year-old matrons, and not a few men. Though bisexual, he preferred the company of females but he would not forego any sexual orgy that might afford him a new experience. Was his insatiable drive for sexual gratification hormonally directed or was he driven by a desire to demean the human spirit? He was indeed cynical and contemptuous of the human race, for he wrote, 'I have seen Folly crowned King of the earth'.

Casanova was no fool. He was a man of boundless interests—he knew the logic of Aristotle, the astronomy of Ptolemy, Latin, a little Greek, and some Hebrew. He studied law but longed to be a physician. In fact, he envisioned the first contraceptive diaphragm. The rind of half a lemon served as a guard around the neck of the womb—a cervical cap. The citric acid enhanced the contraceptive properties of the device because of its spermicidal action. Misanthrope that he was, the oldest medical school in the world—Padua—is proud to claim him an alumnus for he attended classes at the University. Furthermore, as reported in his *Memoirs*, his record of rogueries and amours, against the backdrop of the events of his time, won the attention of historians. Though his book was banned during the Victorian era, interest in this man was revived and biographies dealing with his life and adventures appeared during the decade of the nineteen-twenties by German, French, and English authors. These books relate, just as does his revealing autobiography, how utterly dishonest he was with women and money. This highly intelligent and observant man crowded more adventure, travel, devilry and zest for living into one lifetime than almost any man before or since. Despite his duels, scandals, swindles, banishments, thefts, treacheries, and imprisonments, he was received by George III, Louis XV, Frederick II, Catherine the

Great, and King Stanislaus of Poland. He matched wits with the greatest intellectuals of his time, including Voltaire and Rousseau. How he maneuvered the Pope to present him with the Order of the Golden Spur must remain a triumph of deceit. With equal aplomb, he consorted with pawnbrokers, charlatans, pimps, castrati, ambassadors and cardinals. A delightful and engaging scoundrel with the airs of an aristocrat, he was as much at home in palaces as in the most humble dwelling.

The following vignette is an adaptation from his *Memoirs* to epitomize the day-to-day thinking and activities of Casanova:

Having fled Venice because he was accused of spying, he was now anxious to obtain a pardon and be restored to favor with the authorities. His friends offered to intercede and advised him to live as near as possible to the Venetian borders. He decided to set up his abode in Trieste and since he could not go by land without passing through the State of Venice, resolved to go to Ancona and thence sail for Trieste. On his trip to Ancona, the Jew Mardocheus, shared the carriage. As conversation between them developed, Casanova accused the Jew of being usurious and unmerciful and quoted passages in Hebrew from the Old Testament to prove that Jews were bidden to do all possible harm to the Gentiles. To disabuse him of his mistaken notions, the Jew invited Casanova to take lodgings at his modest but comfortable house where he was warmly welcomed by the family. He was delighted with the arrangement and even with Mardocheus to the synagogue where he noted 'the Jews go to actually pray, and in this respect their conduct is worthy of imitation by the Christians'. After enjoying his accommodations during this extended sojourn, he asked Mardocheus to allow his daughter to keep him company when partaking of his daily snack of *foie gras*. His *Memoirs* record, 'We dined together and I told her that her eyes were inflaming me and that she must let me kiss them'. She did not succumb at first to his blandishments but slowly fell under his spell; ultimately, Casanova seduced her. He was also able to charm his host, for on the eve of his departure for Trieste, Mardocheus prepared a special dinner to show his pleasure in having had so distinguished and learned a gentleman in his home. Casanova, on his part, was filled with gratitude and offered to serve him in Venice should the occasion arise. What a gratuitous offer. What inordinate conceit!

Unlike one with a Don Juan syndrome, Casanova did not need to engage in affairs to prove his virility. His lovemaking was of a different brand. Devising new techniques in the art of love, he enjoyed the sexual encounter as much for the pleasure it afforded him as for the satisfaction obtained in the seductive process itself, and in the mystique of the adventure. Casanova made love under all conditions and circumstances—in beds, on coaches, on staircases, in bathing establishments, and in the open. He also practised sex in any position—lying down, standing, sitting, with one girl or two at the same time, with fake eunuchs, with two men and one girl or two at the same time, with his niece, and with his natural daughter. He was a shameless and unrepentant reprobate, and one might ask: Why his unconscionable behavior? What forces brought him to this state of affairs? Here was a naturally gifted man who would rather be devious than forthright; live by his wits than by honest effort; exploit friend and foe; create mischief; perpetually plot and plan. His greatest joy was to subordinate, subjugate, dominate, seduce, while profoundly basking in his role of arch-deceiver. He suffered from a *libido dominandi*.

What was his background? We must delve into his early years for therein one may find the well-spring of his later behavior. What childhood hurts, adolescent wrongs and frustrations were at the root of this evil force? He was born to a mother who was young, pretty and promiscuous. She was an actress who married at an early age—Jacques was not the child of her husband but the illegitimate son of her director. He was a homely child who was handed over to his grandmother when he was slightly over a year old. A sickly child without appetite or strength, it was said that he looked like an idiot. Was he chided and mocked by other children and scorned by the adults close to him? Did he grow up alienated, unloved, unwanted?

By the time he was fifteen, he submitted to his grandmother's plan to become a *signor abate*, the lowest rung in the ecclesiastical scale. He soon found that wearing his priestly garb gave him an advantage in that he could succeed in his amorous exploits without suspicion. He did not take his 'orders' seriously; for him, religion was not a sacred calling and before long he was in quest of greater fields to conquer.

The passing years gave him a striking appearance. Indeed, the judgement of his witty friend, Prince Charles de Ligne, was that 'He would have been very handsome had he not been ugly'. He compensated for his early unhappiness, parental neglect and abandonment by developing a keen sense of humor, a nimble and observant mind, and a daring which lent him an air of excitement. He developed a personality; he had charisma. Though often without money, he managed by the nature of his dress and manner to appear wealthy.

The question may be asked: Did he ever really fall in love? Yes, with Catarina, a fourteen-year-old girl. He was twice her age when he met her. At first, he actully tried to restrain himself even though she had fallen in love with him. Finally, to make things 'right', he suggested that they be married with God as their only witness. Catarina became pregnant and nearly lost her life when she had a miscarriage. Her father sent her off to a convent where she was to remain until he considered her old enough for marriage. Casanova decided to wait for her release, remaining faithful to a woman for the first time in his life. He passed a most virtuous year, but then he met the nun of Murano and every promise made to Catarina was broken.

Casanova was a conqueror in his own way. Almost every man and woman, in one measure or another, was his prey—to debauch the daughter or wife of his host; to challenge a lesbian; to manipulate a homosexual; to seduce a bride of a week; to 'con' a business associate; to best a political adversary; to swindle a rich widow; to outwit a fellow-intellectual—all were everyday occurrences in his life. He was an impostor who could fit into every society and yet did not belong to any of them. Fear of ridicule haunted him all his life and he based his entire career on a pretense of natural ease. His world was a stage—his life a spectacular; he considered himself the most fortunate of men. His understanding of people's nature brought him many friends, and the number of women who sought him is legion. He reveled in the telling of his *Thousand and One Tales*—a *commedia del arte*. Shortly before his death, on reviewing the events of his life, he was able to say, 'I regret nothing'.

Benito Mussolini

Benito Mussolini with his mistress, Claretta Petacci, was removed by Italian partisans from a German convoy heading for the Austrian frontier. The two were taken to a lonely farmhouse where they spent their last night together. The next day, their captors executed them, brought the bodies to Milan and dumped them on the pavement of the Piazzale Loreto.

The plaza was probably chosen because of its location, with eight avenues fanning out like the spokes of a wheel, making it readily accessible as a gathering place. And the multitudes did come to view the remains of their detested dictator. He had dragged Italy into a war that few wanted, with an ally that none trusted. The frenzied mob hung Il Duce and his mistress head down, suspended by their feet from the girders of a bombed-out gasoline station.

What circumstances brought Mussolini to the pinnacle of power? What inner drives, environmental background, hormonal influences gave the peasant the dynamism to become leader of the proud nation that was Italy?

Benito Mussolini was born on July 29 1883, in a small village near Forli in the North of Italy. His mother, an ardent Catholic, was the village schoolteacher; his father, a staunch atheist and socialist, was the village blacksmith. As a young boy, encouraged by his father, he learned to fight when wronged with a sharpened flint clenched in and protruding from his fist. He got into so many scrapes that his mother packed him off to a boarding school run by priests.

Young Benito grew up embittered, at odds with a society that rebuffed him. He revolted against convention, church, King, and country, and nurtured an obsessional hatred of the rich. At eighteen, with an elementary schoolteacher's certificate, he found employment in a town about a hundred miles from home, but the authorities would not renew his contract as a teacher because of his reputation as a woman-chaser and a misfit. It was in this town that he contracted a venereal disease which he thought to be syphilis. Dismayed, he left for Switzerland, where he took odd jobs to keep alive. Arrested just prior to his nineteenth birthday, he was jailed on vagrancy charges. After leaving prison, a chance meeting with a group of socialists gave him the opportunity to become secretary of the local union of Italian bricklayers working in Lausanne. Speaking at demonstrations and strike meetings, he came to realize that he was a spellbinder. He could mesmerize the discontented workers and electrify a mob.

During his period of growth and development he had many sexual affairs. Starting early in his teens he seduced his cousin and several of her friends. A long series of shabby sexual escapades followed. His amours took place whenever and wherever he found them. His first real mistress was socialist agitator, Angelica Balabanoff, fourteen years his senior. She soon lost interest in him because she felt that his hatred of oppression sprang from a passion to assert his ego.

Banished from Switzerland at twenty-one, he returned to Italy. Contributing frequently to socialist news-sheets, he acquired a reputation as a brilliant but violent and impulsive man. By the age of twenty-six, he had served jail terms for sedition and attempts to incite violence against authority.

In October 1909, he took as his common law wife Rachelle, a barmaid in a wineshop. Benito, in love with this girl, settled down in Forli in charge of a small socialist weekly, and began to intrude into local politics. Rachelle looked upon him as a god-like figure because he was battling for the exploited field-hands and the underprivileged. But one night he staggered home at 5 am smashing all the crockery in the apartment. Rachelle warned him, 'If you ever come home like that again, I'll kill you!' She meant it, and he never did. He rid himself of this vice, but he could not exorcise from his mind his built-in instinct for violence and revolution.

In 1912, he left Rachelle and their little daughter, Edda, in Forli and set out for Milan. There he took over the Milan-based *Avanti*, an ailing Socialist paper. Two years later he was expelled from the Socialist party because he advocated Italy's entry into the war on the side of France and England. Aided by secret monies from France and several Italian industrialists, he started his own newspaper, *Il Popolo d'Italia*. His rallying cry was 'King, Country and Honor'. In late September 1915, he donned the uniform of his country and was glad to get away to confront the Austrians rather than to face Ida Dalser, a shrewish beauty-parlor operator who bore him a son. At the front, while he was exercising, a handgrenade exploded, covering his body with shrapnel. When he recovered, he returned to his editorial desk, pleading for Italy to stand firm and fast against defeatism. The Allies won, but Italy with six hundred thousand dead, almost five hundred thousand wounded, and a colossal war debt gained little. The backlash was bitter disappointment; soldiers returning from the front were shunned by the populace, mistreated by the rank and file, and ignored by the government. Mussolini championed their cause in *Il Popolo*, and his newspaper grew in popularity. On March 23 1919, he saw the chance that would later cast him in his long-cherished rôle of man of destiny. With a handful of friends, he founded the Fascist Party to redress the wrongs, to fight socialism, to defend Italy from Bolshevism. The discontents, the neglected exservicemen, and the disillusioned found common cause. Pockets of the Fascisti sprung up all over Italy, and by 1922 there were three hundred thousand members with their own goon squads— the 'black-shirts'. This rabble was later to prove the model for the brown-shirted stormtroopers that helped bring Hitler to power in Germany. The 'black-shirts' marched on Rome. The King, fearing civil war, allowed this ragged, untrained, undisciplined riffraff to

stream unopposed into the city. A little later, King Vittorio Eman-
uel III invited Mussolini to form a cabinet, and thus a new era for
Italy began—Year One of the Fascist regime.

As a complete novice in government, he found the going difficult. He contrived to do away with the opposition or with any
man who had a following. Matteotti, the leading socialist and a
political threat, was murdered by Mussolini's henchmen. Once he
gained the upper hand, he took over absolute rule. He brought law
and order, abolished the right to strike, started many public works,
and for a time stabilized the economy. He sought to give Italy her
rightful place among nations and was hailed by the people as their
Duce, their guiding genius.

Though he immersed himself deeply in his work, he still had
time for many a tryst. Women were honored to be invited to his
lair; the encounter was usually brief, the Duce hurling them to the
carpeted floor or the cushioned window seat—he was too busy to
waste time on preliminaries. One biographer described him thus:
'All his life, like a stag in rutting season, he had a constant need to
reassert his virility; and he rarely took time to remove his trousers
or his shoes'.

Mussolini, however, believed in moral reforms for others. He
closed fifty-three brothels in Rome, abolished gambling houses,
and shut twenty-five thousand wine-shops. To set an example of
decency and piety, he married Rachelle in a religious ceremony at
Christmas 1925. He was held in adulation by the women of Italy.
A Piedmont school teacher implored him by letter to exercise the
medieval *droit de seigneur* on her wedding night. He sent her a stern
letter. Nonetheless, he continued to have one affair after another.
Angela Civati Cucciati, Cornelia Tanzi, Margherita Sarfatti and
Magda Fontanges were among the more prominent of his mistresses. But one day on his way to the beach at Ostia, there was a
chance meeting with a young girl with whom he became enamored. Her name was Claretta Petacci, the well-educated, smartly
groomed daughter of Dr Francesco Petacci, a senior physician to
the Vatican. As a young girl, Claretta slept with the portrait of
Mussolini under her pillow, much to the chagrin of her father who

looked upon this man as an interloper and demagogue. She worshipped the Duce, and now chance and his cunning threw them
together. He saw her almost every day or wrote frequent love-
letters, always ending on some endearing note like, 'I hope I can be
near you, I would dry them [tears] with my caresses'. Despite his
oft-declared love for Claretta, it was not against his code to have
many other women. Claretta raged with jealousy on learning of
such encounters. Mussolini simply explained that it was his prerogative to exercise his options. Her friends were not averse to keeping her abreast of the box score. She once exclaimed wrathfully to
a friend, 'He has these women seven at a time'. But he convinced
her time and again of his need and his love for her.

There was another quirk in Mussolini's character—his ambiva-
lence toward the Jews. Mussolini basically was not anti-semitic. In
1933 he advised his Ambassador to Germany that 'the anti-semitic
question could turn Germany's friends into enemies'. But after
Hitler's visit to Italy in 1938, there was a change. In 1940, my research fellow, Dr Franco Mortara, showed me a letter dismissing
him from his post as instructor at the University of Bologna. The
letter, in effect, stated that in this seventeenth year of the Fascist
regime, because of the newly adopted Aryan Laws, his tenure was
at an end. The Mortaras could trace their lineage on Italian soil for
over four hundred years. Pope Pius XI, declaring that 'spiritually
we are all Jews', could not convince Mussolini to abandon the
racial laws. Some four hundred Jews found refuge in the Vatican
during those trying times, among them Dr Giorgio de Vecchi
(Rector of Rome University), and the chief Rabbi of Rome. Such
great atomic scientists as Enrico Fermi and Bruno Pontecorvo left
Italy to escape Mussolini's Fascist decrees. Mussolini confided to
the King that 'there are twenty thousand spineless people in Italy
who are moved by the fate of the Jews'. 'Yes, Duce', the King
coolly replied, 'I am one of them'.

My friend Angelo Bettoja of Rome informed me of how his
mother, a Jewess formerly of Seattle, was saved from deportment.
She slept at a different home every night. Another acquaintance,
Giuseppi Block, left Nazi Germany when it appeared that trouble

was brewing for the Jews, and relocated in Milan. When the Germans moved into Italy, he was provided with false identification cards. One night a friend came to his home and pleaded that he head for the Swiss border because the Nazis had discovered the ruse and would arrest him in the morning. He took the advice and found asylum in Switzerland. After the war, he returned to Italy and resumed where he had left off. He is now one of the nation's most respected industralists.

Some months after Mussolini was deposed as head of government and placed under protective custody, he was daringly rescued by Nazi paratroopers and flown to Germany. Several days later he was returned to Northern Italy to set up a Federal Fascist State to carry on the war under German domination and direction. Here Claretta Petacci rejoined her lover, and it was at this time that Rachelle Mussolini learned that she had been his constant companion for almost eleven years. Rachelle understood the inner turmoil and complexities of her husband. She was aware of his many escapades but she shrugged these off as transient affairs that bolstered his ego—affairs of conquest, not love. But Claretta Petacci was another matter—it was as if he had taken a second wife. She sought a meeting with her and during the confrontation called her a whore, predicting that one day she would land in a place called Piazzale Loreto.

About this time, as his troubles mounted, the weary fornicator tried to break off his dalliance with Claretta, but she would have none of it and insisted on following him to the end, even to dying with him. Rachelle's prophecy came true. But why this particular spot in all Milan? Recently, I visited the plaza and made some inquiries, but none could give me the answer. Bemused, I imagined that at some time the place may have been a rendevous for played-out, down-at-heel prostitutes.

One of my Italian colleagues, a radiologist, was interested in learning whether Mussolini had a peptic ulcer, since he so often complained of gastric distress. He informed me that he had read the autopsy report. There was no evidence of an ulcer, only a modest chronic atrophic gastritis; no signs of a glandular disorder; nothing to suggest syphilis. I was able to verify this by studying the necropsy account of Professor C. Mario Cattabeni published July 15 1945. The autopsy findings did not shed light on this innately violent man, this incorrigible womanizer whose sexual exploits were vacuous and meaningless, other than to display his contempt for womankind. This vacillating, indecisive man was swept up in the riptide of history. In his irresolution, he, primarily a socialist, sought later to destroy socialism; he was against his King but later tolerated him; he admired Hitler while secretly despising him; he respected the Jews yet adopted racial laws to make them outcasts; he held his son-in-law, Count Ciano, in great esteem but permitted his execution by the Nazis; he loved women only to demean and subjugate them to his carnal desires. He was indeed a man driven by forces he could not control or understand.

In my search for information about the love-life of Mussolini, many inquiries were made of friends and colleagues in Milan, Florence, Rome, Padua and Genoa. Dr Silvio Dalla Pria, a former research fellow of mine during the years 1967–69, informed me that little was to be found in the Italian press or literature on Mussolini's private life. He explained that the Duce was once a national hero and that the Italian people prefer to remember his strengths and disregard his weaknesses. After all, he did give Italy a new pride; kindled a flame of Empire; gave the common people a workable system of health care; gave employment to the workers and a stabilized wage; and he made the trains run on time. That he brought chaos to Italy was due to his poor judgement in aligning himself with Adolph Hitler. When all honor was lost, a defeated nation realized how badly the people were misled; how blindly they followed the Duce. When his body lay in the Piazzale Loreto, propped up against the white blouse of Claretta Petacci, crowds circled about the bodies in an ugly mood, shouting obscenities, kicking the corpses. The women who but a few months before had idolized this man now impudently spread their skirts and urinated upon his upturned face—the supreme indignity. What an ignoble end for a would-be Caesar! *Sic transit gloria mundi!*

Chapter 7

The nymph and the satyr

*Catherine the Great
and Joseph Stalin*

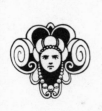

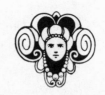

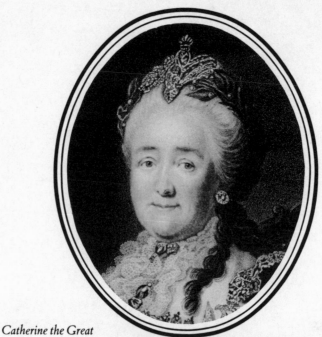

Catherine the Great

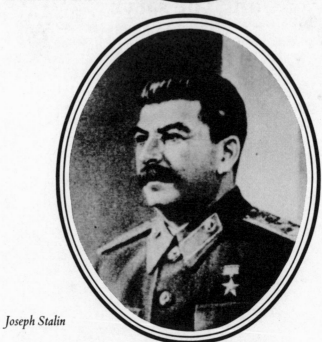

Joseph Stalin

Catherine the Great

Catherine was not her baptismal name; she was not Russian, and though a remarkable woman, was not really great when compared to one of her predecessors—Peter the Great of Russia. Born in 1729 as Sophia Augusta Fredericka, she was the daughter of an impoverished prince of the petty duchy Anhalt-Zerbst in Central Germany. Destiny and determination, sexual unfulfillment followed by sexual gluttony, played important roles in the ultimate design of her place in history.

Time and events were most propitious for Princess Sophia Augusta Fredericka of Anhalt-Zerbst. Reared as the 'poor relation', she showed excellent presence, was well-poised and spirited, though far from pretty. Whether through clairvoyance or vaunted purpose, she, as a mere adolescent, vowed that one day she would wear a crown.

Sophia's ambitious mother made frequent visits to rich relatives dragging her daughter along with hopeful intentions. On one such visit when Sophia was ten years of age, she met a painfully shy boy, Peter Fedorovich, Duke of Holstein-Gottorp, a princedom in Northwest Germany. He, the orphaned son of the elder sister of Elizabeth, Empress of all the Russias, was the sole heir to the Russian throne. A tender feeling developed between the somewhat retarded Peter and the confused and frustrated Sophia.

When the Empress Elizabeth brought the heir-apparent to Russia to groom him for the crown that someday would be his, she initiated a search for a suitable mate. Although Louis XVI of France had a daughter who was under consideration, the King's deep antipathy and distrust of the Russians eliminated any such possibility. Frederick II of Prussia refused to sacrifice his sister and proposed instead his relative—young Sophia of Anhalt-Zerbst. He believed that such a match would not only prove advantageous, but that he would be able to gerrymander and exploit her politically. The Empress accepted the proposal since the Grand Duke Peter had already made known his attraction to Sophia. Accordingly, the young lady was summoned to Moscow to prepare her for marriage. Realizing that her secret aspirations were now within her grasp, Sophia, bright, well-read, innately crafty, was determined to learn the customs, the language, and to accept the religion of her adopted country. At the age of sixteen, she became the Grand Duchess of all the Russias and changed her name to Catherine.

The marriage was a disaster. Peter, poorly educated, ill-mannered, spoiled and inept, proved unequal to the task of matching the spirited, sensuous girl he had married. He was unhappy in his new surroundings for at heart he had remained a German and despised the Russians, while his wife became more Russian than the Russians. But the greatest frustration for Catherine was that Peter was impotent. He never consummated the marriage during the seven years that followed. She began to detest him, and the feeling was mutual. Despite the sexual vacuum, she was not about to fore-sake her chance to wear the crown in the foreseeable future as the wife of Peter III, Emperor of Russia.

Empress Elizabeth, aware of the chaste relationship and disen-chanted with Peter's potential for leadership, decided that some-one else should inherit the throne. The resourceful Elizabeth arranged for one of her courtiers, Serge Saltikov, to seduce the willing Catherine. She became pregnant, miscarried but conceived again and bore a son. The Empress snatched the new-born babe from Catherine's side to rear him in preparation for Kingship. Catherine was ignored and neglected. The Empress Elizabeth had, however, inadvertently opened the floodgates of Catherine's tempestuous passions. She now gave vent to her insa-tiable desire for sexual fulfillment that had been so long denied her. An endless procession of lovers was to follow her to the end of her days, for Saltikov had aroused in Catherine awareness of the joys of sex.

Catherine's court intrigues and her numerous love affairs further displeased the Empress. Catherine was aware of this and strengthened her precarious position by cultivating the brilliant courtiers and the knowledgeable and politically influential men of the realm—many of whom became her sexual intimates. An avid student of political economy and the liberal philosophers of her time and of times past, she was influenced by Voltaire and Montesquieu and read the works of Tacitus and Plutarch. She began corresponding with the outstanding thinkers of the day, such as Diderot and Voltaire.

The Empress Elizabeth sought to keep the Grand Duchess Catherine under her thumb and rule her life. But the younger woman was never happy without a lover. Her *Memoirs* give details as to how she managed to carry on these affairs under the nose of the Tsarina. At times she dressed as a man, often in a male riding habit, and was able to escape from her royal apartment. Also, her lovers visited her dressed as women. Perhaps the idea came from Elizabeth herself: the Tsarina delighted in being hostess at balls where she demanded that guests wear the clothing of the opposite sex. Knowing of this peculiarity probably explains why Count Chevalier d'Eon of France donned feminine attire when he arrived for an appointment with Elizabeth and persuaded her to sign an important treaty with his country. Unfortunately, the French took a dim view of his actions and when he returned to France he found himself in disgrace. In fact, a decree by the French government made it mandatory for him to wear women's clothing for the rest of his life. The word 'transvestism', meaning the abnormal desire to dress in the clothing of the opposite sex, was originally termed 'eonism' although the reason for the Count's action was as much political as his own compulsion to cross-dress.

Count d'Eon gave a graphic description of Catherine whom he observed with interest during his stay in Russia. He described her as being romantic, ardent, and passionate with brilliant eyes which were fascinating and glassy—the look of a wild beast. Her forehead was lofty and he wrote, 'If I am not mistaken, a long and terrifying future is written on it. She is prepossessing and affable, but when she comes close to me, I instinctively recoil. She frightens me'. Probably such a woman would have the same effect on Peter III which could account for his acute dislike of her. But stronger men found her very desirable.

When Peter became the Emperor, he committed every possible folly, groveled before his German hero, Frederick the Great, insulted the Russian Orthodox Church, and threatened to divorce Catherine. But Catherine was not to be outwitted. With political prudence and the support of her many friends at Court, she issued a manifesto in which she claimed to stand for the defense of orthodoxy, and the glory of Russia.

Catherine's current paramour, the handsome soldier Gregory Orlov, hated the Emperor because of his pro-German sympathies and arranged for his brother Alexis to assassinate him; Catherine thus became the sole autocrat of the vast Russian Empire and ruled for thirty-four years. She was in the truest sense the successor of Peter the Great—the monarch who pushed Russia out of her primitive and backward past. A few days before Peter's death, Catherine rode in triumph to Peterhof. She wore a uniform borrowed from a young lieutenant and her hat was wreathed with oak leaves. Beside her rode her intimate friend, the Princess Daschkov, also in male uniform.

What can be said about her reign? Influenced by the liberal philosophers of the West, it was natural that she should start out with the definite intentions of carrying out domestic reforms in Russia through benevolent despotism. She realized that, as a foreigner who usurped the throne, she had to depend on the support of the nobility. She vastly increased their privileges by relieving them from military service and by giving them new powers over their serfs. Serfdom was not mitigated but vastly increased under her rule. The state of affairs was in startling contrast to the humanitarian causes she espoused. The lot of the peasant was worsened and repression greater. While her domestic policies were not those of an enlightened ruler, her foreign policy, aimed at the expansion of Russia, was brilliantly successful. She partitioned Poland, she won the Crimea from Turkey, gaining free access to the Black Sea. She extended the Western boundaries of Russia through diplomacy, aided by her well-chosen ministers and generals. One of these generals and first minister of state was her lover, Potemkin.

Potemkin displayed explosive jealousy and accused her of having fifteen lovers before him, an understatement that she alone appreciated. He could not keep up with her sexual demands and to safeguard his position as first minister actually became her procurer—bringing a stream of handsome young men for her to pamper and make love to. When she tired of them, she sent them away with a gift of land, money, and several hundred serfs. Serfs had become just so much chattel to be used or sold or bartered. The innovative Catherine perfected a foolproof scheme: Potemkin appointed and dismissed thirteen of her lovers in sixteen years; each was examined by the court physician before 'election' to rule out possible venereal disease; each had to be tried out by her principal lady-in-waiting, the Countess Bruce. She acted as *l'éprouveuse*, testing the sexual prowess of the candidate before his appointment. Unfortunately, the Countess found one of the lovers, Ivan Rimsky-Korsakov, so much to her liking that she repeatedly tested the young man after the appointment. On discovery, she was banished.

When Catherine was sixty years of age, Potemkin died. She had replaced him with a handsome twenty-two-year-old lover, Platon Zubov, who, in Catherine's dotage, became complete master of her affairs and an affront to the crown and court. On her death at sixty-seven, her son Paul succeeded her to the throne. Like Shakespeare's Hamlet, he never forgave the murder of Peter III, the man whom he presumed was his father. Paul tried to erase Catherine's name from Russian history.

Catherine was never dominated by her lovers who were the instruments of her policy. It was she who governed, not her favorites—her love-affairs were secondary. She had real political and diplomatic insight and was determined to make Russian society as cultivated as the societies of Paris and Berlin. She had a passion for reading and liked to write. She completed her *Memoirs* and a *History of Russia*, as well as a play. To find time for all her activities she rose at five and worked fifteen hours a day—but at intervals took time off to hide another pregnancy. How many bastards she gave birth to as Empress is unknown. During her marriage to Peter there were two others besides Paul—Princess Anna who was fathered by Count Poniatowski, and Count Alexis Gregorevich

Bobrinsky, fathered by the soldier-politician Count Gregory Orlov.

The scandalous chronicle of Catherine's love-life was the commonplace of all Europe. Polish and Lithuanian refugees from the newly conquered territories spread tales about her disgusting sexual proclivities, the mass orgies, and coupling with animals. The fleeing refugees slandered her with an outrageous fabrication: a bull, suspended over her bed to fornicate with—fell and crushed her to death. The truth is that she died from a heart attack at her writing table after a night filled with love.

The liberal reforms that Catherine had in mind were purely illusory. A century passed before Czar Alexander II (1855–1881) freed the serfs, overhauled the Russian judiciary, improved every level of education and inaugurated representative provincial assemblies—but alas, he was assassinated by revolutionaries who did not want a national consultative assembly. They preferred a despotic anomaly to a tolerable monarchy because they wanted a reason for complete revolution. And so, in time, it happened. In 1917, the Bolsheviks extracted from the adventures of their revolutionary predecessors precisely the same lesson that Alexander's successors did: that the merest hint of liberty leads to sedition and conspiracy, thus making tyranny the only safe government.

It was in this frame of political anarchy that Stalin was able to dominate all of the Russias as the unchallenged ruler of the Soviet Union.

Joseph Stalin

In the Caucasian mountains where Europe ends and Asia begins, Josif Vissarionovich Dzhugashvili was born. He grew up angry, rebellious and embittered. When he rose in status in the Bolshevik Party, he took the name Stalin, meaning 'man of steel'. If indeed he was a man of steel, he had a heart of stone. He turned out to be a most complex and monstrous being. Without a single redeeming feature, he rose to become absolute ruler of the Soviet Union.

Smart, crafty, and shrewd, he possessed an indomitable will to sur-
vive, to succeed, to dominate. This century has known only one
other leader, Adolph Hitler, who equaled him in ruthlessness.
Such men have sex drives that are either strong (Stalin), or weak
and distorted (Hitler). The same personality defects that propelled
them to the top also affected their attitudes toward women. Stalin
dissipated his anxieties and countered his loneliness through frequent sexual relations. Actually, he was sadistic, paranoic, incapable of love or intimacy. His need for sex seemed to
complement and equate with his position of power. Power is the
ultimate aphrodisiac. While Stalin exploited women, they, in
turn, were attracted to him because of his power.

What extraneous forces fashioned such an individual? For
Stalin, the factors were, (1) poverty, (2) the cruelty shown to him
by his father, (3) his defective, shortened left arm, (4) a pock-
marked face, and (5) a small stature.

Joseph Stalin was born in 1879, to a family of former serfs living
in abject poverty near Tiflis in Georgia. His father, a cobbler and a
drunkard, beat his boy frequently and unmercifully. When he was
seven, Joseph fell ill with smallpox which left him with a pock-
marked, disfigured face. His shortened, deformed left arm, said to
be the result of an infection, would seem more likely to have been
due to a birth defect since he also had a defect of the second and
third toes on the left foot. Ever conscious of his size he would
position himself to appear taller. A short stature was a common denominator in the other dictators of his time. Benito Mussolini and
Adolph Hitler were about the same size. Generalissimo Franco of
Spain was slightly under five feet tall. Attila the Hun, the scourge
of God, was even shorter.

At fourteen, Joseph was enrolled in the Tiflis Theological
Seminary by his very religious, widowed mother. Five years later
he was expelled from the Seminary because of poor grades and too
frequent absences from class. Stalin's interest did not lie in his studies for he felt that all the talk about God was pure nonsense—his
concerns were with intrigue and revolution. While in the Seminary, he told on several of his fellow students to the authorities. He

explained that by falsely charging them with subversion they would become better revolutionaries. Soon after his twentieth birthday, he held the only real occupational job in his life—that of a clerk at the Tiflis Geophysical Observatory; his employment lasted less than fifteen months.

Stalin grew up as grim and as heartless as his father—with love for none, with hatred and distrust of all. He was jobless when he joined the Russian Social Democratic Party and began to involve himself in underground activities against the Establishment. It is suspected that he was a double agent working for Okhrana—the secret service police. By betraying certain of his colleagues while enjoying some temporary immunity himself, he was not only able to earn some money, but was able to advance himself while his competition lingered in prison. Nonetheless, his revolutionary activities resulted in his imprisonment or exile for half of his life between the ages of twenty-two and thirty-seven. After he met Lenin in 1907, he became a devoted disciple. However, in 1917, just after the start of the Revolution, the Bolshevik Central Committee granted Stalin membership only on a temporary basis because of 'certain personal traits'. For several years after the Revolution, while Lenin lived, Stalin seemed to revel in being a subordinate. He was all modesty, compliance, and submissiveness. But, according to Louis Fischer, in his book *The Life and Death of Stalin*, 'Lenin's eye pierced the mask of retiring self-effacement and detected ominous signs of grandiose self-aggrandisement'. Lenin warned his colleagues to be wary of Stalin. Lenin wrote in 1922 that Stalin was too rude in personal relations, and abused the power of his office. Lenin was too ill to carry out his plan to expel him. Despite the warnings, Stalin maneuvered by stealth, deception, and cunning to achieve the post of Secretary-General of the Communist Party. He made short shrift of Trotsky, his main adversary and Lenin's rightful heir. The brilliant, well-educated Leon Trotsky was forced to flee. Stalin's fears were not allayed and the long hand of treachery reached across the seas to Mexico where a Soviet agent assassinated Trotsky in his redoubt.

What about Stalin's private life? None dared to write about this side of his life, therefore relatively little is known except that he had married three times and that fidelity was not one of his virtues. He felt there was nothing romantic about sex, that it was a natural function, like eating and drinking. As an atheist, he believed that the feelings of guilt associated with sex and the monastic abstinence in the Christian ethic were obsolete superstitions. Mutual love was to him a decadent Western idea. Only love of the state, the motherland, was meaningful.

Stalin's first wife, Ekaterina, was a simple peasant girl with whom he lived until his mother insisted that he marry her. She died three years later supposedly of pneumonia; some doubts have been raised about her demise, but Stalin is said to have really felt her loss. He told a friend, 'This creature has softened my heart of stone'. Yasha, the one son born to this union was bullied and so harrassed by his father that he once attempted suicide.

Stalin's second wife was Nadja Allilueva, one of Lenin's secretaries. Stalin was obliged to marry her when her father learned that she was pregnant, though she was only eighteen years old at the time. They had two children, Vasily and Svetlana. The first few years of the marriage went moderately well but Nadja could not get accustomed to his crude, rude, selfish, and overbearing ways. She particularly objected to his obscene jokes and to his numerous affairs with government secretaries. After the birth of Svetlana, he no longer shared the marital bed. Sometime later, she separated from him and took the children with her to Leningrad. She was persuaded to return, but found living with her boorish husband intolerable. Early in 1927, Nadja created a stormy scene and threatened suicide if he continued his liaison with a Georgian singer. Another of his mistresses was Yolka Andreyevna, rumored to have borne Stalin a son. Their relationship was once again at breaking point. As Lenin's secretary Nadja had been extremely valuable, but now she had outlived her usefulness. He told her he needed someone to rekindle his spirit and to revive his will to leadership. Offended, she shouted hysterically, 'You are a tormenter, you torment your son, your wife, the whole Russian people'. When she further accused him of usurping the leadership of the

Communist party by dishonesty, purges and liquidations, he seized her by the throat and almost strangled her.

The fifteenth anniversary of the Bolshevik Revolution was celebrated on November 7 1932. The occasion was a dinner given by Voroshilov at his dacha and attended by the leading members of the Party. When Stalin humiliated Nadja at dinner, she stamped out of the room angrily and returned home. A few hours later when Stalin returned, a violent quarrel followed. Next morning, the maid found her dead, sprawled on her bedroom floor with a revolver by her side. Nadja had had a premonition of what might happen. According to H. Montgomery Hyde in his remarkable book on Stalin, it appears that she had confided to a friend, 'I've reached the limit of my endurance. Until now I've been a sort of wife to him, but no more. I'm nothing. The only prospect is death. I shall be poisoned or killed in some prearranged accident'. Whether her death was suicide as Stalin claimed or whether he shot her in a fit of temper will remain conjectural. One thing is certain, Nadja knew too much.

Stalin's third wife was Rosa, sister of Commissar Lazar Kaganovitch. She was a dark-eyed brunette beauty, believed by many, and particularly Nadja, to have been Stalin's mistress for some time. Rosa, a well-educated woman and an accomplished pianist, surrounded herself with poets and writers. She proved too bright and too cultured for Stalin who was bored with her regular musical evenings attended by the intellectuals of the day, including Boris Pasternak, the Nobel Prize-winning novelist. Stalin soon tired of her and divorced her. But Rosa disappeared from the scene and has not been heard of since. She, too, knew too much. Was she liquidated? Did she commit suicide? Was she banished to some forlorn place in Siberia? No one is certain, but this much is known— she was a Jewess and an intellectual. Stalin's antipathy toward Jews and intellectuals was deeply ingrained. Intellectuals who opposed him were in constant jeopardy. For instance, the great Russian author Gorki who wished to leave the country because he was sorely disappointed with the state of affairs, and Stalin in particular, did not make it; he was poisoned and died on June 18 1936.

The Second World War and the dogged resistance of the Russian armies gave to Stalin an aura of greatness. The Soviet propaganda machine and Stalin's sycophants helped to enlarge and embellish his image as a father-figure and heroic idol. Photographs of him in the uniform of a fieldmarshal were distributed throughout the land. He was made to appear taller, thinner, more elegant, according to his own meticulous specifications. The published literature on Stalin always portrayed him as the benevolent father of the country, possessing almost Godlike virtues and qualities. He was pictured just as he liked to see himself, not as he really was. But the cruelty he inflicted on the nation, the millions of dissident peasants that he liquidated because of their opposition to collectivism, the many intellectuals and intransigent army officers that he sent to mental hospitals—these measures could not be forever hidden. The evils of the régime finally came to light, and later Khrushchev declared, 'If he (Stalin) were alive today, I would vote that he should be brought to trial and punished for his crimes'. The Stalin cult died, but unfortunately his repressive measures and the stifling of human rights set a pattern. The Russian people, suffering in silence, have become inured to this way of life. The fact that Svetlana Stalin left her native soil for asylum in America speaks louder than words, for in her books she says little to denigrate her father; one must read between the lines. The three decades of terror and aggression under Joseph Stalin was the theme of Nobel laureate Alexander Solzhenitsyn's book *The Gulag Archipelago*. In 1969, this courageous author wrote, 'We cannot keep silent forever about the crimes of Stalin. For those were crimes committed against millions of human beings and they cry out to be exposed'. The bitter indictment of Stalin is that he ruled Russia for three decades, until his death in 1953, with the permissive cooperation and approval of the people, leaders in science, the arts, and the military. In addition to domestic purges carried out successfully against workers, farmers, intellectuals and Red Army officers, it was Stalin who plotted the public execution of Jews in Moscow in the aftermath of the trumped-up 'doctors' conspiracy' trial in Leningrad.

Through the Soviet Union became a mighty power under

Stalin's stewardship, it is the Russian people who should be complimented. If indeed he raised Russia to greatness, he paid no heed to the millions who were victimized in the process. History will record that among his Russian predecessors he was matched in his savage behaviour by Ivan the Terrible, but in his lusting after sex, he was far outdone by Catherine the Great.

Chapter 8

The madonna–harlot complex

William Ewart Gladstone
and
William Lyon Mackenzie King

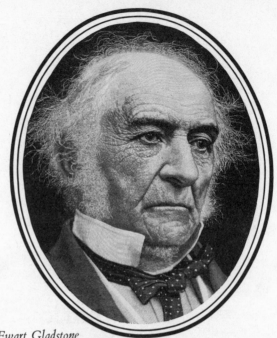

William Ewart Gladstone

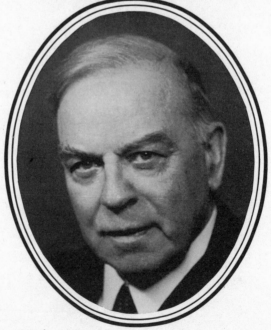

William Lyon Mackenzie King

William Ewart Gladstone

Gladstone was born in Liverpool to middle-class parents who migrated from Scotland. They were devoutly religious and gave their children a rigid evangelistic upbringing. The father, John Gladstone, became a wealthy merchant who traded in West Indies sugar and was involved in black slave labor. He acquired an elegant estate in Scotland where he lived as if 'to the manor born'. In due course, William was sent off to Eton and then entered Oxford where he distinguished himself as president of the Oxford Union. As a young Tory at the University he is remembered for delivering one of the most vehement and eloquent addresses against parliamentary reform. He bitterly opposed the enfranchisement of non-property owners who would dilute the vote of the aristocracy and the wealthy. Gladstone majored in two areas that served him well in later years, classics and mathematics. In 1831, he accomplished the rare feat of winning firsts in both subjects in the same year.

William Gladstone's original intention was to take orders in the Church of England but his Tory friends persuaded him to stand for Parliament. Profoundly religious, he was finally convinced that he could best serve God and humanity by entering the political arena. At age 23, he ran for office. Handicapped by the exposure of his father's involvement in the slave market, he nonetheless won the seat in the House of Commons through his fluency, eloquence and resourcefulness. His extreme conservatism and oratorical skills soon attracted the attention of Sir Robert Peel, who invited him to accept an important post in the Treasury. Later, Lord Palmerston, a staunch liberal, offered Gladstone a cabinet post as Chancellor of the Exchequer. Much to the consternation of his Tory cronies he accepted. Gradually, this able and controversial figure's political philosophy veered from arch conservatism to a most liberal stance. As Chancellor of the Exchequer, he organized the nation's finances and concluded a commercial treaty with England's traditional enemy, France. By shedding the cloak of protectionism and espousing the policy of free trade he vastly improved the economy of the country. Gladstone was the first major politician to bring the issues to the people. In so doing he slowly garnered the love and admiration of the masses and set the stage for the personal triumphs that were to follow.

Benjamin Disraeli, a protectionist who later became the Earl of Beaconsfield, and Gladstone, a free trader, were political rivals. For a time they succeeded each other as Prime Minister. Disraeli, defender of the realm, was a favorite of the Queen but Gladstone, attuned to the *vox populi*, earned only her enmity. In his 60 years in the House of Commons, Gladstone was Prime Minister four times but his strained relationship with Her Majesty never improved. When Disraeli ordered the British Fleet to the Dardanelles as a warning to the Russians to stop their westward expansion, Gladstone opposed the move as a warlike measure and as a threat to peace. Tempers flared throughout the land. The historian and novelist Joyce Marlow captures the divisive feelings in her excellent book, *The Oak and the Ivy*, by quoting two jingles. The Tories sang:

> 'We don't want to fight
> By jingo if we do
> We've got the ships
> We've got the men
> We've got the money too.'

The liberal version was:

> 'We don't want to fight
> By jingo if we do
> The head I'd like to punch
> Is Beaconsfield the Jew.'

Though Disraeli's statesmanship brought peace with honor, it was Gladstone who really averted war. But despite his great accomplishments as a leader, Gladstone was a complex, guilt-ridden man driven by relentless sexual urges. His soul was burdened because of his deep Christian convictions. The extent of the agony that his repressed sexuality brought him was not fully appreciated until 1974 with the publication of the *Gladstone Diaries* by Foot and Matthews.

When did this idiosyncrasy first manifest itself? Gladstone became aware of unusually strong sexual urges while still at Eton. Soon after entering Oxford he wrote in his diary that he was 'the very first of sinners . . . of passions which I dare not name . . . besetting sins which return upon me again and again like a flood. God help me for Christ's sake'. He became engrossed in meeting and conversing with young prostitutes, a pattern that nearly overwhelmed him and became a vital and necessary part of his life. Despite his lust he remained a virgin until his marriage at age 29.

Gladstone was intent on a 'good' marriage. When 23 years of age his proposal of marriage to a lovely, well-born lady was refused. Some time later, he became infatuated with another, only to be rebuffed again. It appears that as a young man he gave the impression of being a solemn, prim and proper person who was regarded by some as a prig. Then, he met and fell in love with Catherine, the comely daughter of Sir Stephen Glynne and the Honorable Mary Neville, who was connected with some of the most illustrious families in England. Catherine recognized in William a potential for greatness, a man who embodied her own ascendant desires. She became active in his political life and was a tremendous asset. Catherine firmly believed in the doctrine of *noblesse oblige*, that privilege entails responsibility. William loved her dearly and she bore him eight children.

Gladstone, who started off as an unbending Tory, ultimately became the standard-bearer of the masses against the more privileged. His favorite work of charity was roaming the streets of London's West End to rescue prostitutes. He brought many home to meet his wife who sympathetically supported him in his imprudent endeavor. Together they founded the House of Charity where wayward women could repair for rehabilitation. The success rate was poor. While Mrs Gladstone's interests were distinctly humanistic, his were of another hue. He enjoyed the pursuit, the vicarious thrill, an excitement he could neither explain nor submerge. Yet Gladstone believed his time spent with prostitutes was a Christian mission, more important than his sexual need. He is the very prototype of the man suffering from a 'madonna–harlot' complex.

For a time Gladstone attempted to sublimate his desires by reading pornography but this pastime did not prove a satisfactory alternative. He could not resist associating with fallen women. Filled with shame at the feelings he entertained during his encounters, he found a temporary remedy for his anomalous behavior. Gladstone started to scourge himself. Flagellation, an old Christian discipline known as *le vice anglais*, proved a deterrent and for several years blunted his preoccupation with prostitutes. He undertook this discipline not as a masochistic form of pleasure but as a form of self-punishment. However, it was not to last and once more he began his nocturnal meanderings. Whatever views were held about Gladstone's attraction to prostitutes, nobody can accuse him of being secretive, nor can anyone prove intimate relationships with his street favorites. In fact, he adamantly refused to be intimidated by two attempts of extortion; he would not submit to blackmail. He had nothing to hide, nothing to fear.

The excitement derived from contacts with prostitutes was a source of anguish. He commiserated, 'Oh that I could live my personal life as I live my public life'. Fortunately, he successfully compartmentalized his life-style and mind-style. His Christian ethics and his iron will prevented him from hurting his beloved wife, impairing his image as a champion of people's rights or his position of public trust. The productivity of his rescue work is best exemplified by the case of the notorious Laura Thistlewayt whose 'house' Gladstone often frequented. She underwent a religious experience in 1852 and with the zeal of a convert became an upstanding and powerful evangelical preacher. This miraculous *tour de force* gave Gladstone great personal satisfaction even though considerable criticism was leveled at him for sponsoring a woman of such dubious background.

Joyce Marlow's intimate biography of the Gladstones, published in 1977, states that the release of Gladstone's private records adds

'. . . a new dimension to our knowledge of a man who more than any other personified English statesmanship in the 19th Century. He helped establish a code of honesty that has become the hallmark of British public service'. My own study of Gladstone's life permits a judgement that his performance in public office was without blemish. Despite many accusations to the contrary and his admitted lust, Gladstone apparently committed adultery only of the heart.

Gladstone was not a hypocrite, nor was he sanctimoniously self-righteous. He did what he had to do to save his sanity and he did it openly. This required great strength and conviction. His personal courage and magnanimity were quite apparent in his struggle for causes that were not necessarily popular but were in harmony with egalitarian and humanitarian principles. As an example, I cite his vote for the admission of Jews to Parliament which irked many of his own constituents. When he died at age 89, he had earned the gratitude of the nation and was referred to as the 'Grand Old Man' by friend and foe. But even in the autumn of his life he continued to serve both God and mammon.

William Lyon Mackenzie King

'There is no doubt, I lead a very double life' wrote W. L. Mackenzie King in his diary (February 13 1898) three months before the death of the man whom he was destined to emulate, William Gladstone. Mackenzie King was later to serve as Prime Minister of Canada for 21 years during his three terms of office. He too suffered from a 'madonna—harlot' complex. He considered his mother the finest, most beautiful and intelligent woman on earth. At an early age, he told her that he would follow in his grandfather's (William Lyon Mackenzie) footsteps and would become Prime Minister some day. He decided on a career in politics. An eerie forecast of events may be fathomed from an uncontrived incident. In 1905 Mackenzie King commissioned J. W. L. Forster to paint his mother's portrait which now hangs in the dining room of Laurier House in Ottawa. Mrs John King is holding a book in her lap,

Morley's *Life of Gladstone*, and it lay open at the chapter 'Prime Minister'. In retrospect, the preternatural confluence of Mackenzie King and William Gladstone may be regarded either as clairvoyance, pure chance, or wishful thinking. The hand of destiny was yet to unfold.

Mackenzie King was born in Berlin (now Kitchener), Ontario, in 1874. His father was a lawyer with scholarly and literary ambitions; his mother was the daughter of William Lyon Mackenzie, former mayor of Toronto and exiled leader of the Rebellion of 1837 aimed at establishing self-government in Upper Canada. Mrs King instilled in her son that it was his destiny to vindicate his grandfather. Mackenzie King had an extraordinary academic career: educated at Toronto University, he later became a fellow of political economics at the University of Chicago, followed by a fellowship in political science at Harvard University. He also studied in London and Berlin. He engaged in social settlement work in the slums of Chicago and this experience tempered his life's outlook—an abiding concern for the underprivileged. He was one of the first Canadian politicians to take an interest in labor and the common man. At heart, he was a humanist; his appearance was one of modesty with a veneer of prudence.

In 1900 King declined an academic post at Harvard to become Deputy Minister of Labor in the newly formed liberal government of Sir Wilfred Laurier. Eight years later he stood as a liberal candidate for Parliament and was elected. He became the first full-time Minister of Labor in Canada. Unfortunately the government fell in 1911 and he lost his seat. In need of money, he accepted a post with the Rockefeller Foundation to investigate industrial relations in the United States. His findings culminated in a pretentious book *Industry and Humanity*. After the death of Laurier the party looked to him for leadership because of his advocacy of social reform without socialism. His opportunity came in 1921 when the liberals gained control. The party chose him as their Prime Minister and a long and eventful career was in the making. Destiny was not to be blunted or denied.

Mackenzie King became one of Canada's leading statesmen

during the first half of the twentieth century. He led the liberal party for 30 years and did much to preserve the unity of the English and French populations, particularly in the difficult times after World War I and during and after World War II. In 1926, at the Imperial Conference in London, King was probably the determining voice in securing the declaration of equality of status for the self-governing nations of the Empire. He led the Canadian delegation to the United Nations Conference. He was fundamentally a liberal who championed social welfare, low tariffs and the rights of the laboring classes. According to the *Encyclopedia Britannica*, 'This remarkable record was achieved by a lonely bachelor, lacking popular appeal, political eloquence or the trappings of a strong leader. His success was a compound of the public mood and a superb capacity for the management of men'. King George VI bestowed the much-coveted Order of Merit on him, the first Canadian ever to receive the award.

What about his double life? None of the half-dozen books I consulted concerning our subject mentions anything remotely suggesting devilish behavior. To all intents and purposes he led an exemplary life. He was a devout Presbyterian who regularly attended church services, sang hymns, read the Bible, prayed for guidance. He was a deeply religious God-fearing gentleman, and for a time conducted religious services for little girls at the Children's Hospital.

King started a diary as an undergraduate student at the University of Toronto and recorded his personal experiences from adolescence to the last days of his life—a span that extended from the closing years of Queen Victoria's reign to the Korean War. It told of his irrational private life which he separated from his rational public world. The document should have been destroyed by his literary executors, since his diary was a confessional. Writing about his sins which brought him shame and deep regret proved a catharsis. The sordid facts came to light in 1977 with the publication of *A Very Double Life* by C. P. Stacey.

Mackenzie King tells of his love of the ladies, particularly the society belles and the daughters of families who were well connected socially and politically. At a reception in Ottawa he spied my wife-to-be, a tall, statuesque brunette. He walked across the room to meet her and in his courtly manner said to her: 'I've never encountered such beauty in any individual.' He indeed was a ladies' man. He was quite popular and had many lady friends but did not allow himself any intimacies. He was attracted to nurses whom he saw as leading selfless lives of service to humanity and to God. He became engaged to a nurse in Chicago who was 10 years his senior. He regarded her as a fine Christian character but when she kissed him ardently on return from a trip to Toronto, he recoiled. He could not equate sexual ardor with a good woman. The engagement was broken. He fell in and out of love several times but seemed psychologically unprepared for marriage.

Early entries in his diary reveal the beginnings of his secret life— 'Went out about 8 and returned at 11:30 . . . saw a little of the dark side of the world which results in my making a firm resolution which, with God's help, I will keep'. Over and over again his diary lists temptation, sin, repentance and tears. He wonders what sort of a man he is to become. He prays for strength, forgiveness, and confesses that he cannot write all that has happened. He records his strolls to seek prostitutes and tells of the restlessness that precedes them. Suddenly we find that King has found a new project—the rehabilitation of young prostitutes. He and a fellow student at the University took up this 'rescue mission' only to become personally entangled.

One of the most poignant entries was made November 19 1896, while studying in Chicago '. . . got into another trap. Cost me $1 . . . wasted time till 5, came home on elevated. I now feel terribly sorry and disgusted at my action. I fought hard against temptation . . . why am I so weak?' The events of November 19 filled him with fear. After his return from spending Christmas holidays in Toronto he consulted a Chicago physician, fearing he had contracted syphilis. He gave up his rescue operations and continued his 'strolls' in Toronto, Chicago, Boston, London, and Berlin, and then in Ottawa. His deep religious beliefs so heightened his feelings of guilt, shame and regret that he became distraught enough

to consult a physician as to his sanity. The doctor gave him 'pow-
ders' to calm his anxieties.

He became quite critical of his compulsive behavior and wrote
in his diary, 'The truth is I am not the man I ought to be. I am the
sort of man I most despise, a hypocrite who plays fast and loose
with life, deals lightly with holy things.' He nonetheless played the
role of the highly respectable public servant who neither drank nor
enjoyed off-color stories. Invited often to address church audi-
ences, he spoke loftily and with deep religious conviction. That he
did not marry was to his credit, for he knew that his passion for
prostitutes precluded any hope of fidelity. Another reason was his
Oedipus complex—five photographs of his mother were on display in his room.

His mother came to live with him during her final illness. He felt
that he ought to stay close by but every once in a while slipped out
to roam the seamy section of the city. One night he went out on
one of his strolls and returned to discover that his mother had
almost died during his absence. That night, he wrote in his diary, 'I
can only feel the goodness of God in sparing her life, and by her
side I consecrate my life anew to purer and nobler service'; his
good resolution was soon broken. He was a complex individual.
His diary records, 'I'm truly a double minded man'. His life was
indeed a contradiction. Though numerous honors were heaped on
him during his lifetime, he actually was inwardly miserable as he
fought a battle which he was unable to win.

*   *   *

We note the sad tale of two great men who toiled for the benefit of
their fellow men and who served God and Country. Each had a
desire to rescue fallen women but in one way or other fell under
their spell. While Gladstone, in all probability, had the fortitude to
resist physical relations, Mackenzie King yielded to his tempestuous emotions. Both were intelligent God-fearing men with
tremendous energies which they exerted for the common good.
Both were victims of a psychological twist—each had high regard

for the sanctity of womanhood but harbored a deep-seated need to satisfy an uncontrollable passion for the company of prostitutes. Prostitutes may appear hard and coarse but often are generous, sympathetic and kind. Perhaps Gladstone and King found in them a degree of empathy, a community of spirit and madonna-like qualities. Was it not said of Mary Magdalene 'Her sins, which are many, are forgiven, for she loved much' (*Luke* 7:47).

Chapter 9

In love
with humanity

*Claude Bernard
and Gregory Pincus*

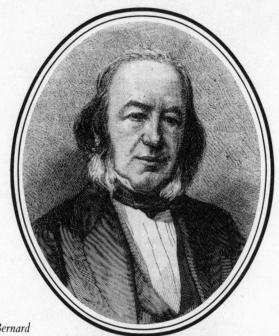

Claude Bernard

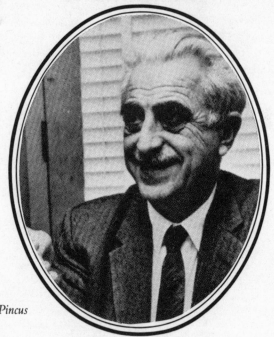

Gregory Pincus

Claude Bernard

Claude Bernard, father of modern-day endocrinology, was born in 1813 on a farm near St Julien (Rhône), France. Little did his friends and family ever dream that this somewhat lackadaisical and unimpressive young man would become France's most illustrious scientist. It was he along with Louis Pasteur who gave France a most enviable position in the newly awakened scientific world of medicine. When Bernard died at the age of sixty-eight, on February 16 1878, he was given a state funeral, the first scientist in France to be accorded such an honor.

Apprenticed to a pharmacist at eighteen, Bernard's employment terminated eighteen months later. His interests lay elsewhere and he was inspired to try his hand at playwriting. He actually earned 100 francs for his comedy, *La Rose du Rhône*. But playwriting was not to be his *métier*. He was advised, 'You have done some pharmacy. Now study medicine.' At twenty-one, he enrolled in medical school. He achieved no great success as a student and some of his instructors regarded him as lazy. He was, however, deeply interested in animal experimentation, ending up as *preparateur* or laboratory assistant to the famous Magendie, the leading physiologist of the day. Bernard progressed rapidly along the line for which he was best fitted—experimental physiology. He believed that 'Those who do not know the torment of the unknown cannot have the joy of discovery' and was always in search of new facts that were in contradiction to widely held theories. He was a seeker of the unknown and toiled diligently in his dark, dank, basement laboratory. His dedication was to lift medical practice from empiricism to a medical science based on truth and facts and not on speculation.

The fortunes of medicine took a new turn with Claude Bernard's concept of the 'internal environment' that brings bodily function into balance. His studies suggested that the liver conserves, stores, and releases sugar (glycogen) according to the needs of the body, keeping blood sugar within normal range.

Early in our civilization it was suspected that the root of some illnesses was a derangement coming from within that was of an intangible and ethereal nature. The Hebrews spoke of body and soul, the Greeks of psyche and soma, the Chinese of the imbalances between the body's ying and yang life-forces. In 1855, Claude Bernard proposed a concept of homeostasis, the *milieu interieur*, which emerged as the touchstone of modern endocrinology. The humoral hypothesis of ancient medical theory conceived health as that condition of the body in which physiological elements are in proper proportion. A disarray of the body humors caused disruption of the harmonious function of various parts of the body. Some four hundred years before the Christian era, Plato introduced the concept of the four humors: blood, phlegm, black bile, and yellow bile. The dominant humor determined an individual's physical and emotional characteristics. His temperament was either sanguine, phlegmatic, choleric, or melancholic. It may well be that the phlegmatic person, dulled by cold phlegm and given to rest and sloth, suffered from myxedema. The choleric man, full of fire and quick to anger may have had thyrotoxicosis. Today we speak of melancholia of the menopausal woman, of personality changes associated with hypoglycemia, adrenal disorders, and parathyroid disturbances. The doctrine of the four humors became the most pervasive concept in medieval medicine and the physician of that era gave a new dimension to the significance of temperament by adding the study of urine (uroscopy) as a guide to diagnosis. The fifteenth-century doctors of the great school of Salerno employed a urine chart of eighteen colors in their attempt to put diagnosis on a sound and scientific basis. The urine glass served as a convenient window for observing the 'humors', for uroscopy was for them the clue to diagnosis.

To reduce excess humor, physicians advised bleeding the patient. For hundreds of years 'bleeding' became a *modus vivendi* and people were bled for diverse and sundry reasons. Bleeding, they believed, restored 'homeostasis' and brought the elements into balance. The phlebotomist came into his own. Actually, barbers performed the procedure at the behest and direction of the physician. This was the wedge that advanced them to the role of barber-surgeon. Incidentally, they moved up in professional status only after one of them cured Louis XIV of a fistula-in-ano. Thanks to a fistula in the royal anus, the barber-surgeon was elevated to the position of 'chyrurgeon'. Bleeding was carried on until late into the nineteenth century. Queen Victoria's consort, Prince Albert, came down with typhoid fever in 1861. Six doctors assisted in his demise by repeatedly bleeding him.

The urine diviners and the phlebotomists were finally displaced by a new breed of scientist. The endocrinologist is the intellectual descendant of the old humoralists, urine diviners, and phleboto- mists. The collection of urine for determination of hormonal levels and the performance of a veritable phlebotomy for a chemical pro- file to determine various electrolytes, lipid fractions, polypeptide and steroid hormones, have in this day become common practice.

Today, the four humors and uroscopy have been replaced by hormonal physiology and modern biochemistry. The products of the glands of internal secretion influence our every living moment—and we are what we are because of our glands, because of our hormonal humors. Shakespeare reminded us, 'We are not ourselves when nature, being oppress'd, commands the mind to suffer with the body'. Osler and Freud understood what Plato, Hippocrates, and Galen knew so well—that mind and body inter- act in the origin and cure of disease. Endocrinologists have not strayed too far from their intellectual forebears—who spoke of the four humors and their influence on man in health and disease. So, it appears, the concept of the four humors was a form of *milieu inte- rieur*, but it remained for Claude Bernard to give it credence through meticulous animal experimentation.

Bernard continued to work prodigiously, and became the grea- test physiologist of the nineteenth century. His monumental book, *Introduction to the Study of Experimental Medicine*, became a classic and is still in use to this day. But the prestigious position he held in scientific circles was not reflected in his home life. His friends had persuaded him to marry the wealthy Marie-Françoise Martin so that he might have some financial security. However, Madame Bernard continually called upon her husband to quit the smelly laboratories and to build a profitable medical practice. She was not willing to forego material acquisitions for intangible honors. His goals were loftier—to help human suffering by penetrating the secrets of bodily disorders and he would not give up his way of life. She did not succeed in her desire to change him but gradually managed to turn his two daughters against him. The domestic conflicts proved tragic and despairing to this great man, eternally absorbed in thought and reflection, and sorely in need of a home where peace and tranquility prevailed. The couple separated in 1869, the year that Emperor Napoleon III called him to become a member of the Senate. The following year, Bernard was divorced from his wife and was also separated from his high political honor by the unfortunate outcome of the Franco–Prussian War of 1870.

His last years were desolate. He was alone, abandoned by his wife and daughters, weakened by repeated bouts of intestinal illness, debilitated by constant and enervating 'fevers'. His morale sank to a very low ebb. It was at this moment that a sweet and affectionate lady entered his life to cheer and calm him, to give him some surcease from his travails. Her name was Marie Sara Roffalovich.

In 1869, at one of his courses at the Collège de France, he caught a glimpse of a well-groomed young woman seated in one of the front rows. He was momentarily stunned by her exquisite beauty and he felt somehow troubled by his emotional reaction. To his surprise, the following day he received a note from her requesting medical consultation. He granted her request, warning that he had not practised medicine in quite some time, but stating he would offer whatever advice he could. From this meeting grew an intimate and endearing relationship—a platonic love that was pure and without guile. Though happily married and devoted to her husband and three children Madame Roffalovich became his confidante and friend. She brought feminine warmth into his lonely and morose life and paid him a thousand little attentions. She met him often, either alone or in the company of her children and her husband. Since Claude Bernard spoke no foreign language (he had never left the soil of France), she was able to be of great service to him by translating scientific German and English articles for use in his speeches and lectures. She became his silent collaborator.

Madame Roffalovich was well born and of Russian ancestry.

She came to live in Paris soon after her marriage. She was a brilliant linguist (Russian, French, English, German, Italian), who was interested in the arts, sciences, and history. She travelled extensively, was a correspondent for the Russian *St Petersburg Journal*, and quite a hostess, having received at her table many renowned men of letters, science, and politics. This talented woman wished to bring some happiness and serenity to a man she venerated and who, in turn, admired her.

Though Bernard had his opponents and detractors, the accolades accruing to him were quite numerous. France honored him with the Legion of Honor; Sweden and Norway with the Order of the Polar Star; England with honorary membership in the Royal Society of London; and Germany with membership in the Academy of Sciences of Berlin. In 1867 he became president of the French Académie des Sciences, and in 1868 was elected to the exclusive Académie Française.

He retired to his native village of St Julien where he lived among his beloved flowers. In constant pain and misery he could only write to his benevolent 'angel' that '*Je continue à vivre, c'est à dire à souffrir*' (I continue to live, that is to say, to suffer.) During nearly nine years of their alliance, Bernard wrote Madame Roffalovich some four hundred and eighty-eight tender missives, an average of one every six days. These letters, which she carefully preserved, form the basis of a book, *Lettres à Madame R.*, prepared by Jacqueline Sonolet. Claude Bernard died as he lived, working, thinking, expounding. He left a heritage of brilliant information which came welling out of his laboratories. Bernard was responsible for the introduction of the scientific method in the art of healing. He laid open the doors of a new science, his methods a beacon for other great scientists to follow. One of these was Gregory Pincus, father of the contraceptive pill.

Gregory Pincus

Gregory Pincus was an unique and extraordinary man. Despite his fame as a scientist, I think of him first as editor, author and poet. Even as a child he exhibited a talent for the written word. Particularly applicable is William Wordsworth's much-quoted line, 'The child is father to the man', for early in grade school he edited the school newspaper, later, the senior class high-school annual. In his senior year at college he was editor-in-chief of the Cornell Literary Review, where a number of his articles and poems appeared during 1923–24.

This capacity for self-expression bourgeoned during his career in which he produced more than four hundred original scientific papers and two books: *The Eggs of Mammals* (1936) and *The Control of Fertility* (1965). His literary and editorial skills found an outlet through membership on the editorial boards of the *American Journal of Physiology and Life Sciences*, in co-editing (with K. V. Thimann and E. B. Astwood) the five-volume treatise *The Hormones: Physiology, Chemistry and Applications*, and as a participant in many scientific symposia. He left to posterity a monument to his prodigious energy—the twenty-three volumes of *Recent Progress in Hormone Research*, which he edited annually until his death in 1967. I am personally indebted to him for a most comprehensive chapter on the Pill written for my book *Ovulation: Stimulation, Suppression, Detection*, published in 1966. As I look back, I now realize that this genteel man could not offend a friend by declining the invitation to contribute. The fact is that he was already a sick man and he undertook this task in the face of mortal illness. What a rare example of courage, hope, duty, and *noblesse oblige*.

Gregory began to write poetry while in high school and continued to do so as a hobby throughout much of his life. Often, early in the morning before leaving for the laboratory, he would scribble a few lines of poetry to his wife, Elizabeth, and pin them to the pillow beside her while she slept. Such tenderness pervaded his whole life-style; the touch of the poet was manifest in his every thought, his every action. Devoted to his wife, he had eyes for no other woman, but for all womankind. He yearned to free them from the fear of an unwanted pregnancy.

Unless a man has trained himself for his chance, opportunities come and go unnoticed. Gregory Pincus did not stumble on the Pill, it evolved, the speck of sand in the oyster that grew into a pearl. Pliny wrote, 'No man possesses a genius so commanding that he can attain eminence, unless a subject suited to his talents should present itself, and an opportunity occur . . .'. The legacy Gregory left to all mankind was a triumph of knowledge, vision and determination. Unlike his ancient forebears who exhorted the Hebrews, 'Be fruitful and multiply', Gregory Pincus, like a latter-day prophet, warned that society had reached that juncture where a calamitous future would await our children's children unless swift measures were taken to curb the population growth. Experience and prescient observation had revealed to him the plight of laboratory rats when too many of them were confined to one cage. Overcrowded, rats become socially maladjusted, irritable, enraged, and eventually begin to devour one another. Food and water, it seems, are then no longer enough. Gregory Pincus saw corollaries where many others saw nothing; yet who would now argue his simple thesis that uncontrolled population growth harbors the dangers of an Orwellian world—an overcrowded world where poverty, famine and socioeconomic instability could ignite war and devastation?

How did his career in biology culminate in this vision and in the development of the Pill?

After his graduation from Cornell University (B.S. 1914), Gregory began graduate studies at Harvard. There he collaborated with his mentor, Dr W. J. Crozier, on studies of the inheritance of physiological traits in mice and rats. In 1927, he was awarded both his MS and ScD degrees. As a Fellow of the National Research Council, he spent several years at Cambridge studying the physiology of reproduction, and at Berlin's Kaiser-Wilhelm Institute pursued his studies in genetics. By 1930, now returned to Harvard, Gregory's curiosity about the developmental sequences leading to certain genetic traits in mammals led to the study of the early stages of rat and rabbit ova. Only six years later came the important—indeed brilliant—discovery that temporary sterility could be induced in rabbits by the injection of estrogens.

In 1939, as professor of experimental zoology at Clark University in Worcester, Massachusetts, he experimented with the induction of ovulation, with ovum transplantation and with parthenogenesis. His preoccupation with ova of mammals and rodents led him to attempt the transplantation of mouse ovaries into rats. Relevant to these experiments is the tale told by Rabbi Levi A. Olan in his 'In Memorium to Gregory Pincus'. The Rabbi relates that one day he wandered into the laboratory and found a pensive Gregory Pincus operating on a rabbit. In innocence, he asked, 'What are you doing?' 'Putting cow's eggs in the rabbit' answered Gregory, matter of factly. 'Why?' 'I'm curious to see what will happen.' As I reflect on that story, I know it was not idle curiosity or feeble humor—no, the future depends very much upon people like Gregory, people who follow intelligent and imaginative curiosities with freedom and with faith.

Pincus's work on mammalian eggs directed his attentions to the hormones that influence reproduction, a research interest that was to dominate his professional life. The decade of the 1940s was largely occupied with explorations of the chemistry and physiology of ovarian hormones.

In 1950, responding to a plea from Margaret Sanger, he was inspired to search for an effective oral contraceptive. With the knowledge that ovulation in mammals could be prevented by estrogens and also by progesterones he began, in collaboration with M. C. Chang, to study other steriods for their ability to inhibit ovulation in the rabbit. The screening of more than two hundred compounds eventuated in the choice of three synthetic progestogens for clinical trial. In collaboration with John Rock, clinical studies with these progestogens were undertaken. In 1956, at the Laurentian Hormone Conference, Rock, Garcia, and Pincus reported that these compounds seemed to suppress ovulation in a group of infertile women they were treating. I was astounded. Following their presentation, I rose ebulliently to discuss their important contribution, proclaiming that they had 'unwittingly given us an excellent oral contraceptive' (*Recent Progress in Hormone Research* (1957), **xiii**,344). Immediately after the session, both Rock and Pincus begged me not to mention the word 'contraception' should the press seek an interview. Contraception was a 'bad' word, and John Rock was not ready to face the ire of the Church fathers for treading the forbidden paths of birth control.

But there was no stopping now, no time for looking back. A new era was here—the Pincus era in science. Pincus made it happen.

Shortly thereafter, in cooperation with Searle Laboratories, Pincus added an estrogen (mestranol) to norethynodrel for greater effectiveness of the compound which was to be used expressly for contraception. In 1960, the Food and Drug Administration gave approval to the marketing of this Pill, now known as the classic or combination Pill. One year later, my own group reported that 100 mg of ethinyl estradiol, administered from day five to day nineteen of the cycle, followed by a progestogen from day twenty to day twenty-four, successfully inhibited ovulation and could be employed in the management of dysmenorrhea, *mittleschmerz*, and severe premenstrual tension, as well as for contraception (*Journal of the Medical Association of Alabama*, (1961) **31**,1). This regimen later evolved into the sequential Pill. Several modifications of the original Pill have been made, and today millions of women throughout the world practice birth control by ingestion of Pills containing an estrogen and progestogen, either in combination or in sequence.

The inhibition of ovulation through the use of estrogens in the management of gynecological disorders was nothing new. Louis Wilson of Brooklyn, and Sturgis and Albright of Boston, employed parenteral estrogens; Haus, Goldzieher and Hamblen, as well as others, employed oral estrogens in cyclic fashion. Greenblatt successfully suppressed ovulation for a whole year in the treatment of membranous dysmenorrhea by the use of continuous oral estrogens, interposing oral progestogens for three days each month to induce regular withdrawal periods. But none of these investigators had the vision to suggest that his regimen might be used for contraception. It remained for Gregory Pincus to focus attention on this important aspect of human need. Pincus had prepared himself for a life devoted to the study of reproductive physiology, and with his knowledge of biology, biochemistry and endocrinology, he was able to grapple with the complexities involved in the hormonal inhibition of ovulation. With deep concern for his fellow man, he set about to find the best means whereby a woman might control her fertility with security and dignity. He was indeed a giant who saw further than his contemporaries. Those of us following his lead are mere pygmies who, standing on his shoulders, may presume to see a little further. Thus far, we have been able to make but mere modifications in his original concept of the physiological interference with conception by hormonal means.

Clark University lost two prestigious and brilliant men when its President and Treasurer attempted to control the research funds awarded certain members of the faculty. In protest, Hudson Hoagland and Gregory Pincus left the institution and established the Worcester Foundation for Experimental Biology in nearby Shrewsbury, Massachusetts, in 1944. They started with a laboratory in an old house, free of the strictures and red-tape of the shortsighted administration that was Clark's. The foundation grew from a single colonial house to a complex of eleven buildings on 139 acres, with a staff of more than three hundred scientists from forty countries. Hudson Hoagland, co-director of the institute with Dr Pincus for twenty-three years, had this to say in his funeral eulogy:

Scientific knowledge to him was the birthright of all mankind, to be fully shared, not merely with his fellow Americans but with all humanity. From the earliest beginnings of the Worcester Foundation, he labored to make it possible for foreign scientists to work and learn in its laboratories and for foreign students to acquire the knowledge and skills that would permit them to return to their homelands and train others. It was his great pleasure especially to train men and women from the industrially underdeveloped countries and thus to export—in their brains, as it were—the possibility of raising the level of well-being in their emerging lands. Even when the illness that was to end his life had.been diagnosed, Dr Pincus gladly accepted calls to journey abroad, often in pain, to lecture and consult with health workers in Europe, India, Latin America, and the Soviet Union.

Another of his endeavors was the organization of the Laurentian Hormone Conferences in 1945. Ever since, two hundred and fifty invited scientists have met annually for a week of formal papers and informal discussions in a stimulating exchange of scientific data as they pertain to various phases of endocrinology. Those of us who have been privileged to attend these Laurentian meetings will never forget the aura that surrounded Gregory Pincus. He was the undisputed leader, the inspiration, the driving force of this loosely-knit organization. He set the high level tone of the conferences and dominated the meetings completely, pleasantly, and effectively. Nor will anyone of us forget Elizabeth, his charming, intelligent wife and constant companion. As the morning sessions ended, she would wait on the balcony of her cottage at the foot of the hill leading from the lecture hall. As a form of greeting she would graciously ask her friends, 'How did it go?' Elizabeth, the queen-bee, held court and presided at the social gatherings.

Gregory and his wife traveled the breadth of the world, organizing colloquia, chairing meetings and committees, participating in conferences and symposia, attending lectures. Dr Abraham White said of him that 'these activities clearly exemplified his belief in the internationalism of science'. He truly became an international figure; I ran into him in Vienna, Milan, London, Lima, Mexico City, and a host of places all over the globe. Through his efforts, I was invited to participate in the International Planned Parenthood Federation meeting in New Delhi in 1959. I was well aware of the energies he had expended in helping to bring scientists from a multitude of countries to share and exchange their knowledge with one another. One day, unbeknown to the rest of the conferees, he slipped quietly away from the meetings to confer with the President of India. He wished to persuade the Head of

State to embark on a plan to control the size of families in over-populated India and to offer his aid. With complete modesty and with no hint of pretension or heroics he told me of this private get-together. It is impossible to overestimate the great role this man has played in education and dissemination of knowledge throughout the world. He was not only a dedicated crusader, he was the ambassador-at-large for endocrinology, the emissary of American science to the world.

What kind of man was Gregory? He was an unassuming man of quiet mien and simple dignity. His face inspired trust, confidence, leadership. His brooding eyes reflected a gentleness and an empathy—the mellowed distillate of a thousand years of ancestral struggle and suffering. He was a compassionate man; gracious and tactful in debate; fair in judgement; resolute; and uncompromising in his search for truths; one who remained forever felicitous to the premise that science must be exploited for the benefit of mankind and not merely as science for science's sake.

The whole world is impoverished by the loss of this man. The message of John Donne is particularly apt,

. . . no man is an island entire of itself; every man is a piece of the continent, a part of the main. Any man's death diminishes me, because I am involved in mankind, and therefore never send to know for whom the bell tolls; it tolls for thee.

His friends have become increasingly aware of the great void brought on by his demise, and are lessened by it. Sir Alan Parkes, in beautiful prose, gave us a word-picture of this man when he wrote:

No one in the history of the human race has lifted the shadow of marital anxiety and frustration so directly from so many of his fellow creatures. I shall remember Gregory Pincus for many things; his passionate interest in science, his vast knowledge, his good fellowship, his generosity to others; but most of all, I shall

remember him for his tremendous contribution to the sum total
of human happiness.

Gregory Pincus will be remembered for his many contributions
to science and medicine. Yet, the true measure of a man extends
beyond his work and the honors bestowed on him. It is also judged
by his heart and spirit—his humanity. The fact that Gregory unsel-
fishly placed the welfare of others before his own is seen many
times over. But never more clearly than during his last months,
when, aware of his illness, he continued with his work even when
plagued by pain and weariness. In a letter to me, his wife wrote:
'His dedication was to science and what scientific disciplines could
do to make the lot of man an easier one. He had a compassion,
understanding, empathy, and a oneness with people. This to me
was faith, devotion, and a manifestation of a true religion.'

The development of the Pill was an outstanding achievement—it might have remained an academic curiosity. With
singular determination, organizational skill and indefatigable zeal,
Gregory Pincus set out to gain world-wide acceptance for this
revolutionary concept in birth control, so that all mankind might
benefit. His long-time friend and colleague, Robert W. Bates,
believed Gregory was able to accomplish this 'not as the domi-
neering salesman . . . but in a quiet unobtrusive way'. If it were not
for Gregory, who can say how long all of the grief and agony
brought on by unwanted pregnancies and the population explo-
sion would have continued. He understood the growing crisis of
his time and was determined to help rectify it, despite unbelievable
road-blocks and considerable hostility.

'The captains and the kings depart', the tide of human events
rolls on with imperceptible change. Few men have influenced the
course of history during or after their lifetimes. Gregory Pincus
was one of these few. He removed the stigma associated with contraception, broke the shackles that kept women enslaved to fear,
and raised the blinds of civilized society, enabling various govern-
ing bodies to take a new look at outmoded abortion laws. He epi-
tomizes the truth of John Steinbeck's theme, 'Man is unique in the

biologic universe because he can climb the ladder of his own achievements and thereby exceed himself'.

Future generations will realize—and be grateful for—this gentle man's impact on the mores and socioeconomics of our times. He has afforded us a keener look at the present and a clearer vision of tomorrow. Like a stone cast into the water causing ever-widening ripples, his work and example have set into motion forces for good that will long endure. Gregory Pincus, affectionately called 'Goody' by his friends, was a good man—in love with humanity.

Epilogue

Indulgence in illicit sex by the famous and infamous is a recurring theme in the history of mankind. David had his Bathsheba. In our own times, the Profumo affair shocked London while pruriency blotted the escutcheon of several Washington Congressmen. One resigned when his secretary, who could not type, confessed in a moment of pique that her duties were sexual not clerical. Another was arrested when he solicited two policewomen who were disguised as prostitutes.

With these exposures, rumors gained currency about the indiscretions and peccadillos of several ex-Presidents. One begins to wonder whether men in politics are more sexually active than the average man and why they are more likely to seek out women of low repute. Dynamic personalities in search of outlets for their boundless energy are the very ones who often seek careers in politics. An intense political vitality may be balanced by an equally intense sexuality.

Over the centuries, society has toyed with a sense or code of sexual values. The lusty sensuality of the Old Testament was earthy. Recall how the Song of Solomon proclaimed with more charm than innocence, 'he shall lie all night betwixt my breasts' (*Song of Solomon* 1:13), or the poet of Proverbs who admonished 'let her breasts satisfy thee at all times; and be thou ravished always with her love' (*Proverbs* 5:19). With the advent of Christianity a change in attitude took place and the Church combined the Jewish ennoblement of sex for procreation (be fruitful and multiply) with the sacred state of chastity (the Greco-Indian ideal of sexual abstinence), placing the greatest possible restriction on sexual feeling—a sort of joyless sexuality. Witness the advice of the Apostle Paul to those who would serve God with the same singlemindedness as he did, 'they that have wives be as though they had none, (I *Corinthians* 7:29) or 'It is good for a man not to touch a woman. . . . But if they cannot contain, let them marry: for it is better to marry than to burn' (I *Corinthians* 7:1,9). The basic rift between spirit and nature which has so troubled the Western world may be traced back to such early Pauline teach-

133

ings. If there is a sexual revolution that is destroying cherished traditions and taboos, if there is greater permissiveness, a new morality, and a 'deterioration' in our mores, then it may be construed as a revolt against an insufferable ethic that sex has to be related to love or procreation alone. Paul's attitudes on sexual morality have increasingly been contested by more liberal theologians.

Today, the Judeo-Christian views on sexual behavior are too often ignored. Permissiveness, promiscuity, mate-swapping, ménage à trios, and voluptuous sex orgies, now extant throughout the land, equal those that plagued ancient Rome. Homosexuality is now regarded as a mild aberration, lesbianism is countenanced, transvestism abounds, and the desire for sexual re-assignment (transsexualism) is no longer an isolated phenomenon.

The values men and women have and should have are merely goals in their struggle to be a little lower than the angels. The common man has learned to expect little from his exalted leaders as exemplars of sexual mores. There has always been one set of rules for the mighty, the famous, and the rich, but it is has always been so. For the power-hungry, the taboos of society are more often 'honored in the breach than in the observance'. Did not Mussolini shut down the brothel houses in Rome, yet hardly a day passed without his seducing some woman? Did not Stalin exhort the masses to a wholesome family life for the sake of Mother Russia, yet unconscionably liquidate at least two of his three wives? Did not Hitler, while glorifying the Aryan race, so degrade his half-dozen female intimates that each attempted or committed suicide?

In the democracies of the world, aspirants to political office and public service are often men of great idealism. They innately have or are conditioned by circumstance to greater aggressiveness, and this property of character may overflow into greater sexual license. Because of idealism and an inordinate reverence for their mothers or their wives, some seek, as Gladstone and many others did, to satisfy their suppressed sexuality by a predilection for prostitutes.

This inquiry into the love lives of the famous and infamous

reveals that power frequently loosens the bonds of discipline. Do they have more compulsive appetites? Is their hold on security so tenuous, so in need of bolstering and constant reinforcement, or is it that the power-drive inevitably produces equally aggressive, unabashed and overbearing sexuality?

(A surprisingly interesting report on the type of men who frequent houses of ill-repute was recently published by Sam Janus and co-workers (A Sexual Profile of Men in Power). Sixty percent of a prostitute's clientele in Washington, D.C., consisted of politicians or political power-brokers.)

The fact emerges that the power–sex syndrome consumes many leaders whom the world reveres or hates. Kings, queens, statesmen, dictators, and politicians often display relentless sexual urges—normal, deviant, or both, to match their power, fame and success. Too often control of the beast within is lost and all the ugly qualities of the human animal come to the fore. Shakespeare, aware of the baser side of man asks, 'What is man? If his chief good and market of his time Be but to sleep and feed? A beast, no more.' And Tennyson reminds us, 'For what are men better than sheep or goats?' There are exceptions: many, many intelligent men and women sublimate their sexual drives, directing their energies to the service of mankind—the result is a love affair with humanity.